KT-528-216

Mental Health Nursing

Case Book

Edited by Nick Wrycraft

Open University Press

Open University Press
McGraw-Hill Education
McGraw-Hill House
Shoppenhangers Road
Maidenhead
Berkshire
England
SL6 2QL

email: enquiries@openup.co.uk
world wide web: www.openup.co.uk

and Two Penn Plaza, New York, NY 10121-2289, USA

First published 2012

A catalogue record of this book is available from the British Library

ISBN-13: 978-0-33-524295-5 (pb)
ISBN-10: 0-33-524295-2 (pb)
eISBN: 978-0-33-524296-2

Library of Congress Cataloging-in-Publication Data
CIP data applied for

Typesetting and e-book compilations by
RefineCatch Limited, Bungay, Suffolk
Printed and bound in the UK by Bell & Bain Ltd, Glasgow.

Fictitious names of companies, products, people, characters and/or data that may be used herein (in case studies or in examples) are not intended to represent any real individual, company, product or event.

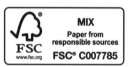

The *McGraw·Hill* Companies

Contents

List of figures and tables

FIGURES

TABLES

Notes on contributors

Geoffrey Amoateng, BEd, RMN, MSc, PGCE is a senior lecturer in mental health at Anglia Ruskin University. Before entering teaching, Geoffrey gained extensive experience in mental health nursing working on both acute admission and psychiatric intensive care units in a medium secure setting, and later as a forensic community mental health nurse. Geoffrey's areas of interest include the development of nursing in pre- and post-registration nursing education, secure mental health care, and the role of culture and how it shapes the understanding and treatment of mental illness among Africans.

Jean-Louis Ayivor is a student mental health nurse and was born in Accra, Ghana, moving to the UK at the age of 14. After completing compulsory education he spent a year in sixth form before pursuing his interest in computer programming and continuing his education in the United States. On returning to the UK, he worked for the NHS, where he developed an interest in psychiatry. Prior to his nurse training, he worked in a low secure unit for 6½ years where he began to grasp the concept of mental health and its complexities. So far, in the final year of his training, he has experienced various placements in a range of mental health settings and acquired new knowledge and skills, which he hopes to implement in his future practice.

May Baker has been a senior lecturer in mental health nursing at Liverpool John Moores University since 2004. She qualified as a mental health nurse in 1994 and worked in acute and community settings. She is a former specialist practitioner and has managed community and in-patient drug and alcohol services. She completed her MSc in Addiction in 2003 and continues to be actively involved with front-line services as part of her role at the university. She has authored chapters on case studies for alcohol – substance use and psychological interventions in drugs and alcohol. Her main teaching interests are alcohol and drug awareness, dual diagnosis and motivational interviewing.

Alison Coad is a qualified occupational therapist and cognitive behavioural therapist. She studied at the University of East Anglia, Anglia Ruskin University and the Kensington Consultation Centre. She has worked for the NHS since 2001, and in 2009 established a private practice. Alison has a wide range of experience in working with children, young people and families, and adults with long-term mental health problems. She also works within an acute hospital setting supporting young people with chronic medical conditions such as diabetes, and as a therapist within an in-patient eating disorders unit in Norwich. Her special interests are the treatment of depression and anxiety disorders.

Hilary Ford is a senior lecturer at Anglia Ruskin University. She has worked in higher education for the past eleven years and currently teaches on the pre-registration programme for mental health nursing. Hilary has a specialist interest in child and adolescent mental health, and she previously taught at both degree and Master's level. Prior to entering higher education, she worked as a community psychiatric nurse in Child and Adolescent Mental Health Services (CAMHS).

Sally Goldspink is a qualified occupational therapist and works as a senior lecturer at Anglia Ruskin University. Her primary clinical interests are in psychosocial interventions and the delivery of individualized, inclusive and collaborative approaches to mental health service provision. This has translated into her academic research which surrounds the development of a contemporary understanding of the student–teacher relationship, particularly within distance learning. Sally has worked closely with academic and practice colleagues to develop distance learning opportunities in order to make education both accessible and relevant for busy practitioners. Sally teaches in both the pre-registration training, and continuing professional development.

John Harrison, BA (Hons), RMN, MSc, PhD, is a senior lecturer in mental health nursing at Liverpool John Moores University. John trained as an RMN in Liverpool and worked as a staff nurse at the Royal Liverpool Children's Hospital with young people suffering mental health problems. He has also worked in the army as a community psychiatric nurse and later as a nursing officer. Following a Master's degree in Nursing from the University of Liverpool, he undertook doctoral research into the perceptions of clinicians towards child self-harm. His research interests are in the areas of self-harm and eating disorders. He is currently involved in a research project examining the concept of body image and disordered eating among gym-using members of the gay community. He teaches on pre- and post-registration nursing programmes and supervises post-graduate research.

Mark McGrath has been in mental health practice for the past 30 years, within the voluntary, public and private sectors. He has been a ward manager for several years and has worked in the fields of community mental health and acute in-patient care, spending the majority of his career to date working within secure mental health care, both within the private and public sectors at low and medium secure levels. Since 2005 he has jointly worked with Anglia Ruskin University and St Andrews Healthcare and in 2010 took up a full-time lecturing post in Mental Health at Anglia Ruskin University. His particular interests are in staff development, both at student nurse and post-graduate levels. He has recently developed several distant learning modules and is a strong advocate for distant learning. His subject specialities are: mental health assessment, risk assessment, forensic mental health and personality disorder (particularly borderline personality disorder). He is a trainer in both the HCR-20 and STAR, and is presently working in collaboration with South Essex Partnership Foundation Trust in developing a Post-Graduate Cert. in Forensic Mental Health.

Michael Nash, MSc, PCLT, BSc (Hons), RMN, FHEA, is currently Assistant Professor of Psychiatric Nursing at Trinity College, Dublin. His academic and research interests include physical health of mental health service users, physical care skills for mental health nurses, mental health service users experiences of diabetes and clinical risk assessment and risk management in mental health nursing. He is also interested in inequalities of health and mental health and speaks Spanish.

Cliff Riordan, RGN, RMN, DPSN, BA (Hons), BSc(Hons), PGCert works as a nurse consultant for Cambridgeshire and Peterborough NHS Foundation Trust, and is an associate lecturer at Anglia Ruskin University, teaching on both pre- and post-registration courses, including modules on recovery and psychosocial family interventions. For the past ten years Cliff has worked in an assertive outreach team with people who experience psychosis, supporting families and carers, and promoting recovery principles in everyday practice. Cliff has also been involved in a number of local initiatives to promote service user and carer involvement in services, and is a member of the Peer Worker Project Steering Group and contributed to the development of an evaluation of the benefits of employing peer workers in mental health settings.

Heather Rugg, RMN, BSc (Hons), Specialist Practitioner, NMC RTQ, began her career in 1998 as a mental health nurse working on a Psychiatric Intensive Care Unit. During this time Heather trained as a specialist practitioner in acute in-patient care, later becoming a case manager in an Assertive Outreach Team working alongside people with severe and enduring mental health problems. Heather remains very interested in both these clinical areas, and maintains strong links with practice. Heather has been a lecturer at University Campus Suffolk since January 2008, and has completed her NMC recordable teaching qualification, and is currently near to completion of the MA in interprofessional education. Heather is the founder and chair of the East of England Regional Mental Health Nurse Programme Forum, and passionate about improving the learning experience of students.

Noel Sawyer is a cognitive behavioural therapist now in private practice providing therapy, training and clinical supervision. Noel trained as a mental health nurse in 1979 at the Maudsley Hospital in Camberwell, London, then completed the ENB 650 course in Behavioural Psychotherapy. Noel has spent his career as a cognitive behavioural therapist developing and managing services in Haringey, north London, and then in Chelmsford, Essex. Noel completed the Post-graduate Diploma in Cognitive Therapy at Oxford University in 1998, an MA in Learning and Teaching at Anglia Ruskin University in 2006 and then an MSc in Advanced Cognitive Therapy Studies at Oxford University in 2008. From 2000 until 2011 he developed and taught the BSc (Hons) and then the MSc in Cognitive Behavioural Therapy at Anglia Ruskin University. Noel has wide experience in treating adults with a wide range of anxiety disorders and clinical depression using various main-stream CBT approaches. His main area of clinical interest is with people who have experienced early traumas and who develop mental health problems. His style of teaching and supervision is the same as his clinical work – developing a shared understanding of the person's learning needs then working in a collaborative manner using didactic, Socratic and experiential methods.

Vanessa Skinner's introduction to the world of mental health care began at the age of 14 when she was admitted into what was at that time termed a 'psychiatric ward'. This experience proved immensely valuable when in 2001, some 35 years later, she qualified as a Registered Mental Health Nurse from Southbank University, earning a special award in recognition of 'The Best All Round Performance on the Mental Health Nursing Branch'. Her next five years were spent developing therapeutic groupwork skills as Deputy Manager of an NHS Day Unit, running therapeutic groups and offering 1:1 therapy while studying for her BSc in CBT, eventually gaining a 1st Class Honours degree from Anglia Ruskin University in 2005. She was later employed by Anglia Ruskin University, both teaching and supervising on the undergraduate and later post-graduate course in CBT. She is registered with the British Association of Behavioural and Cognitive Psychotherapies as a Psychotherapist, Trainer and Supervisor. For the past five years she has been practising as a CBT psychotherapist at Cambridge University Counselling Service, as well as running her own private practice in Ongar, Essex. She is hoping to complete her Master's dissertation in CBT at Hertford University within the next year.

Steve Wood's experience includes undertaking a range of academic roles such as head of department, programme leader and principal lecturer. He has published academic papers and undertaken research on the role of carers of people with dementia, communication frameworks, care management and the care programme approach, mental health and older adults and current provision and future service demand for dementia care. He also has authored a number of publications relevant to the learning and socialization experiences of mental health nursing students. Steve has worked as a community mental health nurse and team leader in older adult mental health care, taken a lead role in organizing workshops on dementia awareness, and has delivered training to a range of professional groups. His specialist interest in older adult mental health, particularly dementia care, has evolved over many years, and Steve is currently a member of a number of dementia strategy groups.

Nick Wrycraft is a Senior Lecturer in mental health with Anglia Ruskin University and has trained mental health students in a range of different clinical roles. Before joining Anglia Ruskin University, Nick worked as a mental health nurse in a variety of clinical settings, and then as research facilitator in primary care. Currently, Nick is completing editorial revisions on his thesis following a successful viva towards a Professional Doctorate in nursing with the University of Essex, and also planning further collaborative writing projects with colleagues. Nick has previously edited: "*An Introduction to Mental Health Nursing*" (2009).

Acknowledgements

I would like to thank my wife Alex and children Emily and Hamish for their support and patience during this project.

Thanks also to everyone who has contributed to this book. I have been very touched by the kindness and enthusiasm of so many colleagues who have very generously given their time and specialist expertise, often at short notice. Finally thanks to Rachel Crookes for commissioning this book, and for her belief and confidence in the project, and to Alex Clabburn, Abigail Jones and McGraw-Hill: Open University Press, for all of your support and assistance.

Introduction
Nick Wrycraft

In recent years the concept of recovery has become increasingly influential in mental health services. Recovery-focused practice is based on the premise that the experience of mental illness is unique for each person, and has a different meaning for each individual. Therefore, people will choose different treatment options, set different goals, and have varying interpretations of what they understand to constitute meaningful change or recovery. In this respect, mental illness is an intensely personal experience.

Recovery contrasts with traditional notions of mental health care, which emphasize diagnosis and the identification of illness, and have been criticized as compounding the stigma, discrimination and social exclusion which people with mental health problems experience in our society. Instead, recovery embraces a positive philosophy which focuses upon the person's coping resources and strengths, and seeks to optimize the full extent of the person's range of positive functioning. In a recovery model, mental health and illness are inextricably linked with all other aspects of the person's life. For people with recurrent mental health problems or for those with an ongoing problem, recovery extends the scope for their potential to live well, and means that mental illness is not something by which the person needs to be defined, limited or labelled.

The case studies in this book have been chosen on the basis of their representing the experiences of individuals, and also in some cases the carers and extended family network of people with mental health problems. Consistent with the notion of recovery, the book proceeds on the premise that fundamental to delivering effective mental health care is valuing the person's individual and personal story, and working collaboratively with them to achieve their preferred goals and aspirations.

The cases are not intended as exemplars of therapeutic intervention, but instead to represent realistic cases with which clinicians deal in day-to-day circumstances, with the same inherent dilemmas and conflicts which are encountered in practice. In this respect it is hoped that the cases will serve as a source to promote discussion, debate and reflection.

In some sections of the book, and across the different sections the same mental health problems are sometimes the focus of more than one case. Consistent with the principles of recovery-based practice the different approaches adopted and interventions used demonstrate the extent to which individual differences of personality, preference, age and other factors exert an influence in how we assess and work with people with mental health problems, and the need to adopt a person-focused rather than illness-focused perspective.

The book is structured into five parts, reflecting a lifespan approach from child and adolescence to older age. Part 1 focuses on child and adolescent mental health, while Part 2 includes cases related to mental health problems which are commonly experienced by adults. Increasingly in recent decades there has been a growing awareness of other mental health problems which adults frequently experience, and Part 3 considers some of these, including alcohol misuse in adults, substance misuse, self-harm, anorexia nervosa and bulimia nervosa.

In Part 4 there are case studies on severe and enduring mental health problems, before we focus on mental health problems in older adults in Part 5.

NOTE ON THE TEXT

A full Glossary is provided at the back of the book. Words that are defined in the Glossary are shown in bold on their first occurrence in the text.

PART 1
Child and Adolescent Mental Health

CASE STUDY 1
Attention Deficit Hyperactivity Disorder (ADHD) in children and young people
Alison Coad

Georgia is 10 and lives with her mum, Emma, her dad, Nick and her younger brother Sam, aged 7. Emma is a teaching assistant at the local first school and Nick is an accountant. Georgia attends the local junior school and will be moving up to high school within the next year. At a recent parents evening, Emma and Nick were concerned to hear that Georgia has been struggling with her schoolwork and has fallen significantly behind in some subjects. There have also been some difficulties in friendship groups and Georgia is often involved in arguments in the playground. On a positive note, her teacher is pleased to report that she is doing exceptionally well at sport.

Emma and Nick have noticed that Georgia has become more and more disorganized over the past 18 months. She has lost many items of school equipment and is often late leaving the house for school and for social events, as it takes her so long to get ready. Georgia is often restless and finds it difficult to concentrate, even on things that she finds enjoyable; for example, it is unusual for her to be able to sit and watch a film through to its conclusion. Emma remembers that she was a lot like this when she was a child, and has not been particularly worried until now. Both she and Nick are concerned about the fact that Georgia is struggling academically but are more worried about the fact that she appears to be having problems making and keeping friends.

1 **Are Georgia's experiences unusual for a child of this age?**

A At the age of 10, a child is developing rapidly – physically, emotionally and intellectually. Physically, the child's strength and co-ordination in undertaking **fine motor** tasks are likely to be increasing at a fast pace. Some children of this age will be entering puberty, with all of the associated physical and hormonal changes. If this is the case for Georgia, it could explain some of the difficulties that she is experiencing in her friendships, as she may be irritable or emotionally volatile.

Cognitive and emotional development is also rapid at this time. Georgia is likely to be demonstrating more independent behaviour and may challenge boundaries. She is likely to be gaining a greater awareness of the needs and feelings of others around her, and of the impact of her behaviour. Her ability to problem-solve and plan ahead should become more apparent at this time but this appears to be problematic for her, both in her school work and in her difficulties in organizing herself which might suggest a developmental problem.

Georgia did not have any problems with academic work before this year and although she was not top of the class, she always managed to meet the expected level of work. When Emma and Nick ask Georgia about what is happening at school, Georgia tells her parents that she is finding it difficult to concentrate and that she often misses instructions given by the teacher.

She has become embarrassed by this and is now hesitant about asking for help as she has been told off on a number of occasions for 'not listening'.

Emma decides to consult her G P, who asks to meet Georgia for an assessment. The G P asks Georgia and her parents to complete a Strengths and Difficulties Questionnaire (SDQ; Goodman 1997) and reviews Georgia's **developmental history**. The G P also spends time talking to Georgia about how she is feeling and how she views the situation.

The SDQ results suggest that Georgia is significantly distressed by her problems at school and also that Georgia's parents have noticed a marked impairment in her functioning recently, particularly her organizational abilities. The G P offers to refer Georgia to a paediatrician at the local hospital for a specialist opinion.

2   **Why would the GP refer Georgia to a paediatrician rather than a mental health service?**

A   Although Georgia is experiencing emotional distress as a result of her difficulties, there is no evidence of **depression** or an anxiety disorder (refer to case studies in this volume for further information). Paediatricians undertake a detailed assessment of a child's development. Poor concentration, poor organizational abilities and restlessness may point to a **developmental disorder** such as Attention Deficit Hyperactivity Disorder (ADHD). It is important that problems such as hearing disorders, epilepsy or thyroid problems are ruled out as symptoms of these conditions can be mistaken for developmental disorders (National Collaborating Centre for Mental Health (NCCMH) 2009). If the paediatrician is satisfied that no significant physical or developmental problems are present, then a referral to a **Child and Adolescent Mental Health Service (CAMHS)** could be considered.

Emma, Nick and Georgia are invited to attend an appointment at the paediatric outpatient department at the local hospital.

3   **How would the paediatrician assess Georgia?**

A   The paediatrician carried out a detailed developmental history by asking a range of questions about Emma's pregnancy. This included questions about Georgia's birth and early development; for example, when she reached significant milestones such as walking, talking and toilet training. Emma explained that Georgia has always been a very 'busy' child, but that this had never been a problem for her parents as they are both very active people. Georgia did not sleep particularly well as a baby, and still finds it difficult to settle down when she goes to bed.

The paediatrician notes that Georgia has been having problems at school and that her academic progress has been affected recently. She also observes that Georgia struggles to sit still during the consultation and that Emma has come prepared with books and toys, which are of limited success in keeping Georgia occupied. Emma admits that this is normal for Georgia and that it has always been difficult to retain her attention for more than around 10 minutes at a time.

Emma and Nick are given some rating scales to complete (Conners' Rating Scales), and are asked to take a separate rating scale into school for Georgia's class teacher. The paediatrician explains that the scales provide a picture of Georgia's behaviour at home and at school, and that this information will be helpful to her in considering what to do next. A further appointment with the family is arranged for two weeks time.

4   **What is the purpose of ADHD rating scales?**

A   Conners' Rating Scales (Conners et al. 1997) have been used in the diagnosis of ADHD since their publication in 1997. They are designed for use in research projects and in clinical settings to identify patterns of behaviour in children and young people, as perceived by their parents and teachers. There is also a self-report form for young people between the ages of 12 and 17 (Conners and Wells 1997). The questionnaires are scored to produce ratings in each of the following areas:

- Oppositional
- Cognitive Problems/Inattention
- Hyperactivity
- ADHD Index

There are also more detailed versions of the questionnaires that can be used where appropriate, for example, if the child or young person presents with symptoms of depression or anxiety in addition to those of ADHD. The questionnaires also help to identify impulsive behaviour that could put the child or young person at risk of harm. A diagnosis of ADHD can increase the risk of substance abuse or involvement in crime (NICE 2008) and a risk assessment is therefore an important part of the review by the paediatrician. For some young people, referral to specialist agencies, such as a youth offending team, may be appropriate.

5   **Are rating scales a reliable way to diagnose problems such as ADHD?**

A   Rating scales, also referred to as **standardized measures**, are used by mental health professionals to assess symptoms of a wide range of conditions including anxiety disorders, depression and ADHD. These scales can be useful in gathering detailed information about the symptoms experienced by patients and/or their families, but it would not be appropriate to rely on them as the sole means of diagnosis. A clinical interview enables the clinician to understand the contexts in which the symptoms occur, and their impact on the patient.

Emma, Nick and Georgia return for the follow-up appointment with the paediatrician. They return the completed Conners' Rating Scales, and the paediatrician reviews the scores during the appointment. Both sets of results indicate that Georgia has significant problems with inattention. There are no obvious problems with **oppositional behaviour**, which corresponds with the accounts given by Georgia and her family, and Georgia's teachers. Hyperactivity scores are low on the teacher's rating scale, and only slightly raised on the parent report scale.

The paediatrician explains that the assessments suggest that Georgia has Attention Deficit Disorder (ADD). Although hyperactive behaviour is often associated with symptoms of inattention and poor concentration, this is not always the case and for Georgia, hyperactivity is only a minor problem. However, it is clear that her symptoms are causing her significant difficulty at school. The paediatrician therefore suggests that it might be helpful to undertake a trial of medication.

6   **What medications would be used in the treatment of ADHD?**

A   In the UK, three drugs are licensed for the treatment of children and young people with ADHD. These are:

- Methylphenidate (marketed as Concerta, Equasym or Medikinet)
- Atomoxetine
- Dexamfetamine

NICE Guidelines (CG72, 2008) suggest that methylphenidate should be considered as the first option for children and young people who do not have **co-morbidities**.

7 **How do drug treatments for ADHD work?**

A Methylphenidate and dexamfetamine are stimulants that affect the **central nervous system (CNS).** They are believed to work by altering brain chemistry, in particular the levels of the neurotransmitters **dopamine** and **noradrenaline** (NCCMH 2009). Both these substances affect mood, movement and concentration. Atomoxetine is not a stimulant drug, but is thought to enhance levels of noradrenaline in the brain.

The paediatrician explains that a treatment trial would involve starting the drug at a low dose and **titrating** this over a period of four to six weeks. During this time, Georgia would be closely monitored for side effects, which can include insomnia, headaches, reduced appetite and nervousness. ADHD medications can also affect growth and it is therefore important that height and weight are checked regularly. The drug can be dispensed in a slow-release formulation, so Georgia would not have to take more than two doses per day.

Emma and Nick are concerned about the prospect of Georgia taking medication and they are not keen to consider this as the first option for treatment. Emma is particularly reluctant as she is very keen on natural remedies and has been researching the positive benefits of omega 3 and 6 supplements for children with attention problems. Emma admits that she is sceptical about the diagnosis of ADHD, as she believes that she suffered similar symptoms to Georgia when she was a child and it did not significantly affect her life. She also raises the point that: 'ADHD has only existed for the last few years. There have always been children with these problems and they didn't have to take medication!'

8 **Is there strong evidence that ADHD exists?**

A Diagnosis of ADHD depends on the opinions of a range of individuals. There is no objective test for the disorder, and it is not always clear which professional service is the most appropriate to care for an individual affected by ADHD. This is one of the reasons why it is so important for ADHD to be managed by multidisciplinary professional teams (NICE 2008). Although diagnosis is not always straightforward, the effects of symptoms reported by children such as Georgia are clear – whatever name these symptoms are given, they can significantly affect functioning and quality of life.

The paediatrician discusses these issues with Emma and Nick, and listens to their concerns about medication. Nick is interested in the idea that these symptoms might be inherited, and wonders if their son Sam might also be at risk of developing problems.

9 **Are ADHD symptoms inherited? Is Sam also likely to be affected?**

A Research suggests that ADHD symptoms are likely to be genetic (NCCMH 2009). Emma reports similar experiences to those currently affecting Georgia, and it would be reasonable to assume that there is an element of **heritability** in this case. Although boys are statistically more likely to develop symptoms of ADHD (Ford et al. 2003, cited in NCCMH 2009), it is by no means certain that Sam will develop symptoms. Emma and Nick ask if there are alternatives to medication.

10 **What other treatments might be helpful for Georgia?**

A The paediatrician is keen to know what Georgia thinks about treatment, and asks her what kind of help she would like. Georgia says that she would like to be more organized, and wants to know if there are things that she can do that might improve her memory. The paediatrician agrees to refer Georgia to the department's psychologist for **cognitive behavioural therapy** (CBT), which can be beneficial in the treatment of ADHD, particularly when inattention is the most troublesome symptom (Kendall 2006). She also suggests that Emma and Nick might benefit from meeting other parents in their situation and recommends a support group organized by the local branch of the ADHD charity, ADDISS (http://www.addiss.co.uk/ accessed 7 August 2011).

Emma asks if it is worthwhile trying food supplements or changes to Georgia's diet. The paediatrician agrees that some parents have noticed significant changes in the behaviour of their children when certain foods are excluded. Research suggests that supplements of essential fatty acids (EFAs) can be beneficial (Hurt et al. 2011) and the paediatrician is happy for Emma to introduce them to Georgia's diet. She advises Emma to keep a food diary and to monitor her daughter's symptoms over the coming months. A follow-up appointment is arranged for three months time.

At the follow-up appointment, Georgia reports that she has felt more settled at school recently. She has joined the netball team and has played for her school, which has improved her confidence and introduced her to new friends. Georgia is not sure if her concentration is any better, but her sessions with the psychologist have helped her to become more organized through using a diary and reminders on her mobile phone.

Emma and Nick have attended two meetings at the local ADHD support group, and have had the chance to talk with parents who have chosen to accept medication for their children. As a result of this, they are less opposed to the idea of medication as a result, but tell the paediatrician that they would like to wait and see how Georgia manages the transition to high school before they decide what to do next. They have adjusted Georgia's diet, as the food diary revealed that foods with artificial colouring seemed to aggravate her symptoms. Georgia continues to take EFA supplements daily, as several parents at the support group have reported good results on this regime.

Emma asks the paediatrician if Georgia will continue to have symptoms of ADHD when she is an adult.

11　Does ADHD carry on into adulthood?

A　Adults can be diagnosed with ADHD, and those diagnosed in childhood have a strong chance of at least some of their symptoms persisting into their twenties and beyond (NCCMH 2009). NICE (2008) suggest that approximately 2 per cent of the adult population worldwide are affected by ADHD.

Georgia is offered a further review appointment in 12 months time.

REFERENCES

American Psychiatric Association (2000) *Diagnostic and Statistical Manual of Psychiatric Disorders*, text revision. Washington, DC: APA.

Conners, C.K, Sitarenios, G., Parker J.D.A., and Epstein, J.D. (1997) The Revised Conners' Parent Rating Scale (CPRS-R): factor structure, reliability, and criterion validity, *Journal of Abnormal Child Psychology*, 26(4): 257–68. Available at: http://dx.doi.org/10.1023/A:1022602400621 (accessed 6 August 2011).

Conners, C.K. and Wells, C.K. (1997) *Conners-Wells' Adolescent Self-Report Scales*. Toronto: Multi-Health Systems, Inc.

Goodman, R. (1997) The Strengths and Difficulties Questionnaire (SDQ). Available at: http://www.sdqinfo.org/a0.html (accessed 6 August 2011).

Hurt, E.A., Arnold, L.E. and Lofthouse, N. (2011) Dietary and nutritional treatments for attention-deficit/hyperactivity disorder: current research support and recommendations for practitioners. *Current Psychiatry Reports.* Available at: http://www.ncbi.nlm.nih.gov/pubmed/21779824 (accessed 7 August 2011).

Kendall, P.C. (ed.) (2006) *Child and Adolescent Therapy: Cognitive Behavioral Procedures,* 3rd edn. New York: The Guildford Press.

NCCMH (National Collaborating Centre for Mental Health) (2009) *Attention Deficit Hyperactivity Disorder.* British Psychological Society and The Royal College of Psychiatrists.

NICE (National Institute for Health and Clinical Excellence) (2008) *Attention Deficit and Hyperactivity Disorder: Diagnosis and Management of ADHD in Children, Young People and Adults.* Clinical Guideline 72. Available at: http://www.nice.org.uk/nicemedia/live/12061/42107/42107.pdf (accessed 7 August 2011).

Appendix: DSM-IV Criteria for ADHD

I. Either A or B:

A. Six or more of the following symptoms of inattention have been present for at least 6 months to a point that is disruptive and inappropriate for developmental level:

Inattention

1 Often does not give close attention to details or makes careless mistakes in school-work, work, or other activities.
2 Often has trouble keeping attention on tasks or play activities.
3 Often does not seem to listen when spoken to directly.
4 Often does not follow instructions and fails to finish schoolwork, chores, or duties in the workplace (not due to oppositional behavior or failure to understand instructions).
5 Often has trouble organizing activities.
6 Often avoids, dislikes, or doesn't want to do things that take a lot of mental effort for a long period of time (such as schoolwork or homework).
7 Often loses things needed for tasks and activities (e.g. toys, school assignments, pencils, books, or tools).
8 Is often easily distracted.
9 Is often forgetful in daily activities.

B. Six or more of the following symptoms of hyperactivity-impulsivity have been present for at least 6 months to an extent that is disruptive and inappropriate for developmental level:

Hyperactivity

1 Often fidgets with hands or feet or squirms in seat.
2 Often gets up from seat when remaining in seat is expected.

3 Often runs about or climbs when and where it is not appropriate (adolescents or adults may feel very restless).
4 Often has trouble playing or enjoying leisure activities quietly.
5 Is often 'on the go' or often acts as if 'driven by a motor'.
6 Often talks excessively.

Impulsivity

1 Often blurts out answers before questions have been finished.
2 Often has trouble waiting one's turn.
3 Often interrupts or intrudes on others (e.g., butts into conversations or games).

II Some symptoms that cause impairment were present before age 7 years.
III Some impairment from the symptoms is present in two or more settings (e.g. at school/work and at home).
IV There must be clear evidence of significant impairment in social, school, or work functioning.
V The symptoms do not happen only during the course of a Pervasive Developmental Disorder, Schizophrenia, or other Psychotic Disorder. The symptoms are not better accounted for by another mental disorder (e.g. Mood Disorder, Anxiety Disorder, Dissociative Disorder, or a Personality Disorder).

Based on these criteria, three types of ADHD are identified:

1 ADHD, *Combined Type*: if both criteria IA and IB are met for the past 6 months.
2 ADHD, *Predominantly Inattentive Type*: if criterion IA is met but criterion IB is not met for the past six months.
3 ADHD, *Predominantly Hyperactive-Impulsive Type*: if criterion IB is met but criterion IA is not met for the past six months.

Depression in children
Alison Coad

Jade is 14 years old and lives with her mother and father. She is the younger of two children. Her older sister has recently graduated with a first-class degree, and has obtained a good job in London. Jade's parents are high achieving professionals – her mother is a senior nurse and her father is a lawyer. They are keen for Jade to pursue a career as a doctor.

Six months ago, Jade transferred to the local girls' grammar school as her parents felt that the local state high school was 'not academic enough' for her. Jade was not keen to make the move as she had a good group of friends at her old school, and was very involved in the school drama society. However, she agreed to the move to please her parents, and because she knew that she would have to achieve very high grades at GCSE and A level in order to gain a place to study medicine.

Since transferring schools Jade has become increasingly withdrawn and irritable at home. She finds it very hard to get up in the morning and she is struggling to keep up with the amount of homework that she gets. She has put on weight and has started to worry a great deal about her appearance, especially her teeth, as some of the girls at her new school have been making remarks about Jade needing a brace. Because the workload at her new school is so much more intense, she has stopped socializing with her old friends at the weekends and has lost touch with them. Her parents have recently received a letter from school asking them to attend a meeting with Jade's head of year as Jade has been absent without authorization on three occasions over the last month. When her mother questions her about this, Jade breaks down and tells her mother that she is very unhappy at her new school and has missed some days because she cannot face going in. She has also become so upset about the remarks about her teeth that she is afraid to talk to other girls in case they notice them and make fun of her. Jade's mother is shocked to hear how unhappy Jade is and is worried about the amount of weight that Jade has gained. She arranges an appointment with the family GP, who thinks that Jade might be depressed and so refers her to the local Child and Adolescent Mental Health Service (CAMHS) for an assessment.

1 **What are the symptoms of depression in a child or adolescent?**

A Children and young people demonstrate similar symptoms to those of adults suffering with depression, that is, persistent low mood, changes in appetite and sleeping patterns, increased irritability and impaired concentration.

2 **How common is depression in children and adolescents?**

A Cartwright-Hatton (2007: 11) notes that 'in one recent ... study of children in Britain, ... nearly 1 per cent of children were found to be clinically depressed'. Allen and Sheeber (2009), citing Costello et al. (2006), highlight the fact that rates of depression rise from

2.8 per cent in children under 13 to 5.6 per cent in adolescents. Although these figures sound small, they suggest that in a high school with 1000 pupils, there are likely to be 50 who are clinically depressed. The 2001 Census (Office for National Statistics 2004) revealed that nearly 80,000 young people in the United Kingdom suffer from severe depression.

Jade and her mother attend an initial appointment at the local CAMHS clinic, where a nurse therapist, John, undertakes an assessment. John is interested to know about Jade's family history, and learns that Jade's mother and maternal grandmother suffered from depression in their twenties. Jade's mother was treated with **anti-depressants** and recovered within 12 months, but her grandmother has continued to experience episodes throughout her life.

3   **What causes depression in young people? Is depression hereditary?**

A   There is some evidence to suggest that children of depressed parents are more likely to become depressed themselves (Tompson et al. 2009) but it is important to consider this information in context. There are a range of factors that may make a young person susceptible to depression, and genetics and heredity should be seen as factors within a complex picture. Developmental factors, including puberty and the maturing of the brain, combined with psychosocial factors such as family events, academic demands and peer pressure, interact throughout adolescence. For Jade, critical incidents appear to have been her transfer to a new school, increased academic pressures, and the loss of a pleasurable and rewarding activity (drama). Additional factors may be her family's high expectations of her, and her increasing anxiety about her personal appearance.

4   **What other diagnoses might be considered when assessing Jade?**

A   It is not unusual for a young person with a diagnosis of depression to have a co-existing diagnosis of another psychiatric disorder (Seeley and Lewinsohn 2008). This is known as co-morbidity. Jade's account of her worry about her appearance may point to **body dysmorphic disorder (BDD)**. Distress resulting from a perceived physical defect can be a sign of BDD, an anxiety disorder which can be extremely debilitating (Veale et al. 1996).

Other disorders which are frequently diagnosed concurrently when depression is identified are substance abuse disorders, eating disorders and **obsessive compulsive disorder (OCD)**. It is also important to be aware of symptoms such as excessive energy and unusually elevated mood, as these can signify a different kind of depressive disorder (bipolar disorder). **Bipolar disorder** is likely to be a long-term diagnosis and is more likely to be treated with medication, as manic episodes may involve impulsive, and therefore risky, **behaviour**. Jade does not present with any symptoms of this kind but John remains alert to the possibility of body dysmorphic disorder.

John asks to speak with Jade on her own for part of the assessment, and he learns that Jade has been feeling so low in mood recently that she has started to **self-harm** by cutting herself on her upper arms. The cuts are superficial but John can see that there are some old scars. Jade admits that she started to cut shortly after starting at her new school. She tells the nurse that she has been feeling so distressed at school, especially since the teasing about her teeth started, that she sometimes feels that she cannot cope. One evening after a particularly bad day at school, Jade was so upset that she used the blade from a pencil sharpener to cut her arm. She found that cutting helped to relieve some of her tension and has continued to use it as a way to manage distress. She is always careful to cut in an area where her mother will not see it.

5 **What are the key issues for the professional in managing self-harm?**

A Self-harm can take a variety of forms, including cutting, burning, overdoses and drug and alcohol abuse. A thorough **risk assessment** should always be a part of an initial assessment, and this should be clearly documented within the patient's notes. Suicidal **risk** is obviously very important and can be assessed using a standard assessment such as the Beck Intent Scale, which enables the professional to gather key information in a systematic way (Beck et al. 1979). The risk assessment should be reviewed on a regular basis. In the case of a young person who is known to be self-harming, monitoring should be a part of every appointment and any significant concerns discussed with the young person and communicated to the multi-disciplinary team. If risk is deemed to be too high to manage on an out-patient basis, an in-patient admission may need to be considered.

Fortunately, Jade's presentation does not warrant referral to an in-patient unit but there are **risk factors** that John needs to take into account when assessing her needs. Jade does not want her mother to know about her cutting as she is fearful that her mother will be angry.

6 **Is John obliged to tell Jade's mother about her self-harm?**

A The rules of confidentiality between a young person and their therapist should be explained as a part of the assessment process. John had explained to Jade and to her mother that matters discussed in session would remain confidential within the CAMHS service, unless issues pertaining to risk called for consultation with other agencies (such as social services). During his discussion with Jade, he is required to make a professional judgement about the level of risk posed by Jade's cutting, and whether or not it is necessary to disclose this to her parents in order to ensure her safety. He then needs to balance the question of risk with that of Jade's **engagement** in the therapeutic relationship. John assesses the extent of Jade's self-harm and agrees that he will not disclose this information to her parents provided that she is able to take responsibility for keeping herself safe. This includes minimizing the risk of infection by keeping the wounds clean and covered, and ensuring that she does not cut any deeper than the existing cuts. John also needs to ensure that Jade is aware of the dangers of cutting and of the fact that cutting on certain other areas of her body may pose more of a risk of serious harm. He also provides an information sheet providing a list of alternatives to self-harm, including drawing on the skin with red pen, pinging rubber bands against the wrist and rubbing the skin with an ice cube (National Self-Harm Network 2007).

John believes that Jade is significantly depressed and arranges an appointment for her to see the team's psychiatrist, as he thinks that Jade might benefit from medication. He also offers a follow-up appointment within a week, in order to ensure that Jade is closely monitored and supported.

7 **What medications might be prescribed for children and young people suffering from depression?**

A NICE guidelines recommend the use of **fluoxetine** for young people between the ages of 12 and 18 who are experiencing moderate to severe symptoms of depression, and who have not responded to 4–6 sessions of individual psychotherapy (NICE Guideline CG28, September 2005). If fluoxetine is not tolerated, or is ineffective, either citalopram or sertraline may be considered as second-line options. These medications are all **selective serotonin reuptake inhibitors (SSRIs)**. As the NICE guidelines point out:

> Fluoxetine does not have a UK Marketing Authorisation for use in children and adolescents under the age of 18 at the date of publication (September 2005) ... [however] unlicensed medicines can be legally prescribed where there are no suitable alternatives and where the use is justified by a responsible body of professional opinion.
>
> (Royal College of Paediatrics and Child Health 2000, cited in
> Quick Reference Guide to CG28, p. 13)

Fluoxetine may be used 'cautiously' in children between the ages of 5 and 11 (Royal College of Paediatrics and Child Health 2000, cited in Quick Reference Guide to CG28, p. 13).

The psychiatrist assesses Jade and agrees that anti-depressant medication would be helpful. However, Jade is not keen to take medication, stating that she needs to 'sort this out for herself'.

8 Can depression be treated without medication?

A Recent studies focus on the ongoing debate about the role of medication in the management of depression in children and young people. Research studies such as ADAPT (Adolescent Depression Antidepressant And Psychotherapy Trial; results published in 2007) and IMPACT (Improving Mood with Psychoanalytic And Cognitive Behavioural Treatment – results expected in 2016) aim to provide new data which can be used to inform clinical decisions. These trials are both **randomized control trials**. The ADAPT trial results suggested that the addition of cognitive behavioural therapy (CBT) made very little difference to outcomes for young people with depression also treated with an SSRI (Hazell 2007). The IMPACT trial seeks to explore this issue further. At the time of writing, the NICE guidelines recommend that young people should not be offered medication without psychotherapy (NICE 2005: 7).

There is evidence to suggest that CBT alone can produce changes within the brain that are similar to the effects of anti-depressant medication (see, for example, Linden 2006). It is therefore appropriate to offer psychotherapy as a stand-alone treatment if this is agreed between the patient and their healthcare professional.

Jade asks what other treatments might help her. The psychiatrist explains that talking therapy might suit Jade – the clinic offers psychodynamic therapy, cognitive behavioural therapy and systemic therapy.

Jade explains that she would like to continue to meet with John as she found him to be very understanding. She does not have a particular preference about the type of therapy but she is very clear that she would like one-to-one therapy. She is not keen for any of her family members to be part of her sessions. John uses a psychodynamic approach and agrees to offer Jade six sessions in the first instance. The Glossary provides further information about the differences between the types of therapy offered in CBT, **psychodynamic therapy** and **systemic therapy**.

Jade attends six sessions with John and, together, they are able to identify that Jade's problems are mostly related to her parents' high expectations of her. It emerges that she wants to work in theatre, and is not interested in becoming a doctor. She discloses that she is 'too scared' to discuss this with her parents as she believes they will be disappointed and angry. The difficulties she has experienced settling into her new school have made her feel much more isolated and have led to comfort eating and avoidance of situations that make her feel more vulnerable. The fact that Jade's mother is very critical of her daughter's weight has been the cause of difficulties between mother and daughter since Jade was a small child. John encourages Jade to explore her feelings about her parents and to think about ways in which she can begin to communicate her feelings to them. Jade agrees that her parents can be invited to a session to help her to articulate some of her concerns in a neutral environment.

John agrees that he will continue to offer Jade regular appointments in order to help Jade to develop some strategies to improve her self-esteem. She also agrees to attend a walking group organized by the clinic's occupational therapist, who is conducting research on the benefits of physical exercise for the treatment of depression. The research has been developed in response to the findings of the review of the current NICE Guideline (CG28), which noted that 'areas to consider in future updates of the guideline [included] physical/biological treatment of depression encompassing exercise therapy, sensory, dietary and nutritional interventions either individually or as part of a multimodal intervention' (NICE 2011).

Jade remains a patient at the clinic for 18 months. She is discharged when she is no longer self-harming and her mood has improved sufficiently for her to feel able to manage without therapeutic support.

REFERENCES

Allen, N.B. and Sheeber, L.B. (2009) The importance of affective development for the emergence of depressive disorders during adolescence, in N.B. Allen and L.B. Sheeber (eds) *Adolescent Emotional Development and the Emergence of Depressive Disorders.* Cambridge: Cambridge University Press.

APA (American Psychiatric Association) (2005) *Diagnostic and Statistical Manual of Mental Disorders,* text revision. Washington, DC: APA.

Beck, A.T., Kovacs, M. and Weissman, A. (1979) Assessment of suicidal intention: the Scale for Suicide Ideation, *Journal of Consulting and Clinical Psychology,* 47(2): 343–52. doi: 10.1037/0022-006X.47.2.343 (accessed 24 July 2011).

Cartwright-Hatton, S. (2007) *Coping with an Anxious or Depressed Child.* Oxford: Oneworld Publications.

Hazell, P. (2007) Depression in adolescents, *British Medical Journal,* 335: 106. http://dx.doi.org/10.1136/bmj.39265.581042.80 (accessed 24 July 2011).

Linden, D.E.J. (2006) How psychotherapy changes the brain: the contribution of functional neuro-imaging, *Molecular Psychiatry,* 11: 528–38. Available at: http://dx.doi.org/10.1038/sj.mp.4001816 (accessed 24 July 2011).

National Self-Harm Network (2007) *Distractions that Can Help.* Available at: http://www.nshn.co.uk/downloads/Distractions.pdf. www.nshn.co.uk (accessed 17 July 2011).

NICE (National Institute for Health and Clinical Excellence) (2005) *Depression in Children and Young People.* Clinical Guideline CG28. Available at: http://www.nice.org.uk/nicemedia/live/10970/29858/29858.pdf (accessed 24 July 2011).

NICE (National Institute for Health and Clinical Excellence) (2011) *Review of Clinical Guideline CG28 – Depression in Children and Young People.* Available at: http://www.nice.org.uk/nicemedia/live/10970/53353/53353.pdf (accessed 24 July 2011).

NIMH (National Institute of Mental Health) (2011) Teenage brain: a work in progress (Fact Sheet). Available at: http://www.nimh.nih.gov/health/publications/teenage-brain-a-work-in-progress-fact-sheet/index.shtm (accessed 24 July 2011).

Office for National Statistics (2004). Available at http://www.ons.gov.uk/ons/guide-method/census/census-2001/index.html (accessed 13 March 2012).

Seeley, J.R. and Lewinsohn, P.M. (2008) Epidemiology of mood disorders: implications for lifetime risk, in N.B. Allen and L.B. Sheeber (eds) *Adolescent Emotional Development and the Emergence of Depressive Disorders.* Cambridge: Cambridge University Press, pp. 33–55.

Tompson, M.C., McKowen J.W. and Asarnow, J.R. (2009) Adolescent mood disorders and familial processes, in N.B. Allen and L.B. Sheeber (eds) *Adolescent Emotional Development and the Emergence of Depressive Disorders.* Cambridge: Cambridge University Press.

Veale, D., Boocock, A., Gournay, K., Dryden, P., Shah, F., Willson, R. and Walburn, J. (1996) Body dysmorphic disorder: a survey of fifty cases, *British Journal of Psychiatry*, 169: 196–20. doi: 10.1192/bjp.169.2.196 (accessed 24 July 2011).

FURTHER READING

Bellani, M., Dusi, N., Yeh, P.H. et al. (2010) The effects of antidepressants on human brain as detected by imaging studies: focus on major depression, *Neuro-Psychopharmacology and Biological Psychiatry.* Available at: http://dx.doi.org/10.1016/j.pnpbp.2010.11.040 (accessed 24 July 2011).

British Association for Counselling and Psychotherapy website. Available at: http://www.bacp.co.uk/seeking_therapist/theoretical_approaches.php (accessed 25 July 2011).

Goodyer, I., Dubicka, B., Wilkinson, P., Kelvin, R., Roberts, C. et al. (2007) Selective serotonin re-uptake inhibitors (SSRIs) and routine specialist care with and without cognitive behaviour therapy in adolescents with major depression: randomised controlled trial, *British Medical Journal*, 335: 142. Available at: http://dx.doi.org/10.1136/bmj.39224.494340.55 (accessed 24 July 2011).

Office of the Children's Commissioner (2007) *Pushed into the Shadows: Young People's Experiences of Adult Mental Health Facilities.* Available at: http://www.chimat.org.uk/resource/item.aspx?RID=56424 (accessed 24 July 2011).

Young Minds. Available at: www.youngminds.co.uk (accessed 17 July 2011).

APPENDIX: DEFINITION OF DEPRESSION

The NICE Guidance (2009) identified the *Diagnostic and Statistical Manual* (DSM) definition of depression, where at least one of the key symptoms needs to be present in sufficient severity for most of every day for 2 weeks together with 5 of the other features in sufficient severity for most of every day over 2 weeks.

Key symptoms

1 Persistent sadness or low mood, most of the time.
2 Markedly reduced interest in all or almost all activities for the majority of the time and loss of interest/pleasure – nearly every day.

Other symptoms

• Appetite and unplanned weight loss (5 per cent of total body weight within a month, or the equivalent) or weight gain.
• Disturbed sleep – **insomnia** or **hypersomnia**.

- Psychomotor agitation, or reduction of activity most of the time.
- Fatigue and a lack of energy and interest most of the time.
- Feelings of worthlessness, or guilt most of the time.
- Reduced, and a slowed-down ability to think, concentrate or make decisions most of the time.
- Recurrent thoughts of death or suicidal ideation most of the time.
- Somatic symptoms, for example, aches and pains.

James is 14 years old and has been taken to see the G P by his mother, who is concerned about his mood and his behaviour. Recently he has been refusing to travel to school on his own and when his mother encourages him to walk, he often returns to the house after a few minutes, appearing tearful and anxious. When in school, he has been missing lessons and staff have been concerned as there have been some occasions when he has gone missing. James's mother has tried to talk to him about what is troubling him but he finds it very difficult to express his worries verbally. This has led to tensions at home. James's mother also reports that when James is worried about something he can become angry and aggressive.

James is academically talented and is studying for 13 G C S Es. He lives with his mother and older sister. His father suffered from clinical depression and committed suicide four years ago. James's G P decides to refer him to the local Child and Adolescent Mental Health Service (C A M H S) for assessment.

1 **How would you recognize symptoms of anxiety or depression in children and adolescents?**

A Symptoms of anxiety and depression differ between individuals and the presentation in young people can be very different to that in adults. For example, depression in young people can lead to high levels of irritability and temper outbursts. Anxiety often leads to outbursts of temper due to high levels of adrenalin ('fight or flight' hormone) and the resulting state of hyper-vigilance, which leads the person to pay excess attention to events which, for other people, pose no threat.

The **DSM-IV** (American Psychiatric Association 2000) provides definitions of the range of different types of anxiety disorder. These are:

- **generalized anxiety disorder (GAD)**;
- panic disorder;
- panic disorder with agoraphobia;
- **phobias**;
- **obsessive compulsive disorder (OCD)**;
- **post-traumatic stress disorder (PTSD)**;
- separation anxiety;
- childhood anxiety disorders.

Each category is defined by specific symptoms with different recommended modes of treatment. It is therefore important to understand what kind of anxiety disorder your patient might have.

In James's case, his symptoms include fear of being out in public, fear of being judged and a tendency to isolate himself. This would fit with a diagnosis of social anxiety but there may be other diagnoses that would also apply to James, for example, panic disorder.

In order to understand James's symptoms more clearly, and to establish a baseline of the severity of his current symptoms, it can be helpful to use a standardized measure such as the Beck Youth Inventory. This is a self-report questionnaire with five separate sub-scales. A questionnaire is useful if the client finds it difficult to express their worries and is a good way to obtain a lot of detailed information without interrogating the client. This is particularly relevant when working with children and young people, as the experience of being interviewed by health professionals can be very daunting.

James and his mother attend an assessment appointment with a cognitive behavioural therapist from the CAMHS team. James appears extremely shy and uncomfortable and so the therapist has to work very carefully to engage James in the assessment process.

2   **What factors need to be considered when undertaking a mental health assessment with a child or an adolescent?**

A   Any mental health assessment must take into account factors such as risk – to self, to others, or from others. Assessment of suicidal ideation is particularly important. This is especially true in James's case, as his father's suicide has left the whole family in a position of fear and anxiety about any risk of self-harm. In addition to this, it is important to gather personal information such as the client's age, their social circumstances, and the impact of symptoms on day-to-day activities, including work or school. Meeting a mental health professional can be daunting for a client of any age and can be very uncomfortable for young people. It is therefore especially important to work on engaging a young client and in building a safe and trusting therapeutic relationship. One of the most important factors is clear definition of the confidential nature of the relationship between therapist and client. The initial meeting with the client needs to establish the rules of confidentiality very clearly, and must include an explanation of any circumstances that would require the therapist to breach confidentiality.

3   **What if a child or young person tells the therapist something but does not want that information to be shared with their parent(s)? Do parents have a right to know?**

A   It is often appropriate to provide the opportunity for the young person to speak to the therapist alone. The presence of parents or carers can sometimes inhibit a young person, either because the young person is embarrassed or fearful of the consequences of disclosure. There may be key information – for example, the young person's use of drugs or alcohol, or episodes of deliberate self-harm such as cutting – that would not be disclosed in the presence of parents or carers, and that the young person would not wish their parents to know. Of course, some of these issues might come into the category of significant risk. If that is the case, a sensitive judgement would need to be made about who needs to know what is happening. The key issue is the safety of the young person but it is important that the therapist works collaboratively to ensure that the young person feels heard and that they have choices.

Giving the young person choice – about whether they answer questions, where they sit in the room, who is present in the session with them – can encourage engagement. It can also be useful to make a clear statement early on in the assessment about the length of the appointment, what will happen during the session, and what will happen after the session. It is also important to be clear about the limits of the help that can be offered. Maintaining a professional relationship, while offering warmth and containment, is an important balance, particularly with vulnerable clients such as young people.

James's mother is very concerned that James may be more likely to suffer with a mental health problem because of his father's history.

4 **Are mental health problems inherited?**

A Taking a family history, including a **genogram** (a family tree) and details of any physical or mental health difficulties within the extended family, is an important part of the overall assessment. A family history of anxiety or depression may predispose a young person to these conditions; that said, mental health problems can affect any individual, regardless of genetic factors.

The CBT therapist learns that James has become increasingly anxious about school since starting his GCSE courses. The academic standards at his school are very high and he gets a lot of homework. His mother has noticed that he is becoming anxious about leaving the house and is not socializing with his friends as much as he used to. His sleep has become erratic and he finds it very difficult to get to sleep. As a consequence, he is often very tired. He is spending more and more time alone in his room playing on computer games.

The CBT therapist decides to ask the team psychiatrist to assess James as she thinks that he may be in need of some medication to help to reduce his levels of anxiety.

The psychiatrist assesses James and diagnoses a clinical level of anxiety. She decides that he could benefit from medication, which she prescribes. She arranges to review him in a week's time.

5 **What medications might be prescribed for a young person suffering from high levels of anxiety?**

A Selective serotonin reuptake inhibitors (SSRIs) are recommended as treatment for adults with anxiety disorders (NICE 2007; 2011). There has been a lot of debate in the literature around the use of SSRIs for young people (see, for example, Hodes and Garralda 2007). A significant concern has been the question of a link between the use of SSRIs and increased suicidality in young people and a lot of work has been undertaken on this question (Whittington et al. 2004).

NICE guidelines (2005: 11) state that 'doctors may make decisions based on the individual clinical needs of a child or an adolescent to use these products for the treatment of depression or anxiety'. A prescription of fluoxetine at a dose of 10 mg daily can help to settle severe anxiety symptoms.

6 **What other interventions could be beneficial for James in respect of his anxiety symptoms and his difficulty sleeping?**

A Anxiety management strategies can include applied relaxation training, breathing exercises, and cognitive techniques that help the individual recognize the links between thoughts and physiological symptoms of anxiety. Imagery can be a useful technique, for example, in the form of a guided relaxation, where the client may be talked through a scenario that they find relaxing such as lying on a warm beach. This can be helpful for individuals who find it difficult to 'switch off' from their thoughts. Simple tips about sleep habits (referred to as **'sleep hygiene'**) are often recommended by healthcare professionals. Avoiding daytime naps, taking regular exercise, and paying attention to caffeine intake are standard sleep hygiene tips. Watching television and computer use (including electronic games) before bed can cause sleep disturbance and should therefore be monitored and reduced if necessary.

7 **Why does the psychiatrist need to review James? How often would she need to see him after this?**

A When prescribing psychiatric medication, it is the prescribing doctor's responsibility to ensure that the client is reviewed on a regular basis. It is the doctor's duty of care to ensure that any side effects are manageable and that the young person and their carer have access to a professional who can answer any questions.

In As noted above, there is some concern that fluoxetine may increase the risk of suicidal activation and it is obviously very important that patients should be aware of this and other possible side effects. The prescribing doctor should monitor James closely for symptoms such as agitation and nausea.

James's mother is keen for James to receive some psychological support to help him understand his difficulties and to learn techniques to manage them.

8 **Can CBT be helpful for children and adolescents suffering from anxiety disorders?**

A Cognitive behavioural therapy is recognized as an effective treatment for children and adolescents diagnosed with a range of anxiety disorders. There is a considerable amount of published evidence to support this, with the first randomized controlled trial using CBT to treat anxiety disorders in children taking place in 1994. A wide range of trials have been conducted since then, with some reporting diagnosis remission rates of over 60 per cent (Stallard 2009).

The CBT therapist offers to meet with James on a weekly basis. He asks for his mother to be present during his appointments as he feels uncertain about talking about the issues that are worrying him.

9 **Is it helpful for a child or adolescent to be accompanied by a parent during therapy sessions?**

A The question of whether a parent should accompany a young person in CBT sessions varies according to the needs of the young person, and the nature of their relationship with their parent(s). For younger children, parental involvement might be necessary to help the child to feel safe enough to engage in therapy. Parents can also become co-therapists, learning techniques such as **graded exposure** to feared situations in order to practise them at home. However, in certain circumstances, parental involvement may hamper the progress of therapy, for example, if the parent is highly anxious. If the problem is particularly complex or pervasive, for example, in some cases of obsessive compulsive disorder (OCD), parents can become deeply involved in the completion of OCD rituals. This feeds into the **maintenance cycle** – that is, the process that keeps the problem going (see Figure 3.1, James's **formulation**, for an explanation of the maintenance cycle). Sometimes the young person can be inhibited by a parent's presence, and might withhold important information, especially relating to risk-taking behaviours such as self-harm. It is therefore important to balance all of these factors. Stallard (2009: 17) suggests that 'the extent and nature of parental involvement in CBT will vary. At a minimum, parents should be involved in regular review meetings.'

10 **How does the therapist engage with James?**

A The therapist helps James to work out which situations are most difficult for him. She asks him to identify the thoughts that go through his head when he is feeling anxious, and

Predisposing factors

Father's history of depression

Tendency to perfectionism (e.g. high academic standards)

Not a 'verbal' child – finds it hard to talk about feelings

Key events (sometimes described as critical incidents)

Father's suicide

James's beliefs

Unknown situations are frightening and dangerous

James's assumptions (life rules)

If I am frightened, then I will be humiliated

If I am not in control, then the worst could happen

James's feelings (emotional and physical)

Scared, anxious, hot, shaky

James's behaviours

Avoid situations that might be frightening – hide

Consequences
Social withdrawal and no chance to test out fears – so fears grow, negative thoughts and feelings are reinforced, and James becomes more withdrawn (the vicious circle, or maintenance cycle)

Figure 3.1 James's formulation

what kinds of physical and emotional responses occur in these situations. James finds it very difficult to put these experiences into words and so the therapist uses imagery and age-appropriate language to support James in his expression of his fears. Through the use of drawings and analogies, James describes symptoms of rapid heartbeat, blushing, 'jelly legs' and sweaty hands. These symptoms occur when James is in any situation where he feels as though he is the focus of attention, for example, when a teacher asks him a question in front of the class. He also worries a great deal about getting into trouble, for example, when he forgot his homework he became so anxious at the prospect of being reprimanded by the teacher that he did not feel able to attend the class and hid in the library.

Cognitive behavioural therapists gain an understanding of the client's problems by developing a formulation (see Figure 3.1). A very important part of the formulation is the maintenance cycle – that is, what keeps the problem going. For James, avoidance is the behaviour that perpetuates his symptoms of anxiety and it is therefore necessary to work out ways to help him to face the situations that are causing him such distress.

11 **What techniques could the therapist use to help James to deal with his symptoms of anxiety?**

A Key techniques to help James to tackle his anxiety might be:

- **Psycho-education** about anxiety and how it can affect us.
- Keeping an 'anxiety diary' – writing down a daily record of situations that provoke anxious responses. Recording things in writing is a common technique in CBT.
- Graded exposure to feared situations – tackling fears in a step-by-step way, breaking the problem down into manageable stages. This helps individuals to tolerate anxiety in a gradual way.

- Behavioural experiments – ways to test out assumptions that are unhelpful, for example, the assumption that 'If I forget my homework and the teacher shouts at me, I will become so upset that I will lose control and embarrass myself.' Behavioural experiments can help clients to find out whether feared consequences are likely to occur.

12   How many sessions of therapy might James need?

A   CBT is a time-limited treatment, and NICE guidelines suggest varying packages of treatment according to diagnosis (see www.nice.org.uk: Summary of cognitive behavioural therapy **interventions** recommended by NICE, NICE n.d.). For children and young people with moderate to severe depression, NICE recommends individual therapy over a period of at least three months. James suffers from a mixture of symptoms of anxiety and depression and it would be reasonable to expect him to need between 12 and 20 individual sessions of CBT.

13   How does the therapist measure James's progress?

A   CBT therapists routinely use standardized measures such as the Beck Youth Inventory as a means of monitoring the progress of their patients. These measures are questionnaires that the patient is asked to complete on a regular basis throughout a course of therapy – usually at assessment, halfway through treatment and at the end of treatment. For adults, the Beck Depression Inventory (BDI) or the Beck Anxiety Inventory (BAI) might be used. These scales can also be used for young people at the discretion of the therapist.

14   Will James be more likely to experience problems with anxiety in future because of his history of anxiety as an adolescent?

A   Young people who have experienced depression or anxiety may be more vulnerable to experiencing similar problems in the future. It is therefore important to include relapse prevention work within the course of therapy offered. This can include revision of techniques, encouraging the young person to be aware of early warning signs (such as avoidance of certain situations, or sleep difficulties) and ensuring that the young person knows how to seek help in future.

James feels that his symptoms have improved sufficiently to allow him to attend school daily (and remain in lessons), make his own way to school and to ask for help from staff when he is feeling particularly anxious. His mother reports that he is much calmer at home, and that arguments have greatly reduced. Scores on the Beck Youth Inventory have reduced to within normal range. The therapist therefore arranges a follow-up appointment in three months, to review progress and address any unresolved difficulties.

REFERENCES

American Psychiatric Association (2000) *DSM-IV–TR*, text revision. Washington, DC: APA.

Hodes, M. and Garralda, E. (2007) NICE guidelines on depression in children and young people: not always following the evidence, *Psychiatric Bulletin*, 31: 361–2.

NICE (National Institute for Health and Clinical Excellence) (2005) *Depression In Children and Young People: Identification and Management in Primary, Community and Secondary Care.* Clinical Guideline CG28. Available at: http://www.nice.org.uk/guidance/CG28 (accessed 22 May 2011).

NICE (National Institute for Health and Clinical Excellence) (2007) Clinical Guideline 22 *Anxiety: Management of Anxiety (Panic Disorder, with or without Agoraphobia, and Generalised Anxiety Disorder) in Adults in Primary, Secondary and Community Care*. Available at: http://www.nice.org. uk/nicemedia/pdf/CG022NICEguidelineamended.pdf (accessed 13 March 2012).

NICE (National Institute for Health and Clinical Excellence) (2011) Clinical Guideline CG113. Available at: http://www.guidance.nice.org.uk/CG113 (accessed 22 May 2011).

NICE (National Institute for Health and Clinical Excellence) (n.d.) http://www.nice.org.uk/usingguid-ance/commissioningguides/cognitivebehaviouraltherapyservice/summarycbtinterventions.jsp (accessed 29 May 2011).

Stallard, P. (2009) *Anxiety: Cognitive Behaviour Therapy with Children and Young People*. London: Routledge.

Whittington, C.J., Kendall, T., Fonagy, P., Cottrell, D., Cotgrove, A. and Boddington, E. (2004) Selective serotonin reuptake inhibitors in childhood depression: systematic review of published versus unpublished data, *The Lancet*, 363(9418): 1341–5. DOI: 10.1016/S0140-6736(04)16043-1 (accessed 22 May 2011).

FURTHER READING

Beck, A.T. (1993) *Beck Anxiety Inventory*. San Antonio, TX: Pearson Education Inc.

Beck, A.T., Steer, R.A. and Brown, G. (1996) *Beck Depression Inventory II*. San Antonio, TX: Pearson Education Inc.

Beck, J.S., Beck, A.T. and Jolly, J.B. (2005) *Beck Youth Inventories*, 2nd edn. San Antonio, TX: Pearson Education Inc.

Stallard, P. (2002) *Think Good, Feel Good: A Cognitive Behaviour Therapy Workbook for Children and Young People*. Chichester: John Wiley & Sons, Ltd. Available at: http://www.rcpsych.ac.uk/mental-healthinfoforall/problems/anxietyphobias.aspx (accessed 22 May 2011).

WEB RESOURCE

http://www.patient.co.uk/showdoc/125/ (accessed 22 May 2011).

Childhood generalized anxiety disorder (GAD)
Hilary Ford

Sara is a 14-year-old girl who has become increasingly anxious since the separation of her parents ten months ago. Sara's dad, Simon, has moved abroad and she only sees him during the school holidays although they share many interests including swimming and music. Simon has been a constant source of support and reassurance throughout Sara's life.

Sara has recently experienced difficulty in concentrating at school and appears excessively anxious. She has uncontrollable worry about everything from schoolwork, to friendships and feeling different in the relationship with her friends since her dad left home. Sara worries in case her dad becomes seriously ill, and worries about the world recession and the impact this will have on her dad's business abroad

Sara is often tearful, complains of feeling constantly restless, and has muscle tension and cannot get to sleep at night because of her worries. Jan, Sara's mum, sits with her, listening to her repeat her worries until she eventually falls asleep. Jan is struggling to cope.

Sara feels tired in the mornings, does not look forward to school and is concerned that she will be too tired to do her schoolwork, or will miss the school bus and be told off for being late. Jan and Sara have regularly been arguing over trivial issues and becoming impatient with one another.

Sara is academically able, but now showing deterioration in her schoolwork. She is normally a very sociable and fun-loving person, but has become very serious and withdrawn and recently refused to go on a school camp, believing her friends would not want her there. Sara has also started avoiding sleeping over at friends which she previously used to enjoy.

During frequent visits to the school nurse Sara received **counselling** to talk about her feelings. However, the decline in her mental health has led the school nurse to refer Sara to the local Child and Adolescent Mental Health Services (CAMHS) out-patient department for a more specialized assessment and help. Sara and her mum attended an assessment meeting with a CAMHS nurse.

1 **What considerations might be made before and during the early stages of the assessment to address any concerns Sara and Jan might have about the meeting?**

A A leaflet was sent to Sara and Jan, together with the letter confirming the appointment, providing general information about the clinic and an explanation of the service. When asking children or young people about their physical symptoms, it is often helpful to use simple language appropriate to the age and functional level of the person (DoH 2008).

Sara and Jan were greeted and welcomed on arrival for the assessment and the CAMHS worker made the introductions and then explained their role and the areas on which the assessment would focus. The CAMHS worker also asked Sara and her mum their views on the reason for the referral and their expectations and hopes for the meeting. This demonstrated a collaborative working approach which actively involved Sara and her mum and empowered them while ensuring that their concerns and priorities were addressed. Issues regarding confidentiality and consent were then explained, and it was stated that if there were concerns over Sara's safety, it would be necessary to share information with other professionals.

As part of the assessment, Sara's developmental history was considered, which included her past health and functioning. A detailed account was taken of the milestones of her physical and emotional development, including motor, sensory and cognitive development. The CAMHS worker also asked Sara and her mum whether she had experienced any significant health problems. Any previous behavioural or emotional difficulties such as anxiety were also considered, for example:

- separation anxiety
- simple phobias
- social phobias
- generalized anxiety disorder
- panic disorder.

These conditions were specifically focused on, as the first three have a higher prevalence among younger populations, with the latter two being associated with adolescence (Goodyer 2005). In Sara's case, she had no previous developmental problems, except for mild separation anxiety in early childhood.

When the CAMHS worker moved on to discuss Sara's current difficulties, it appeared that her performance at school and her friendships were significantly affected. Her relationship with her mum has also become strained as Jan no longer knows how to help Sara and feels helpless. Both Sara and Jan want their relationship to work again. Sara would also like more contact with her dad and to be able to resume her activities and social life but finds the anxiety significantly debilitating.

Sara described constantly feeling anxious at school and home, and lacking confidence in peer relationships and leisure activities, to the point that she is unable to control her worries. She is beginning to lose contact with friends and is socially withdrawn, for example, recently refusing to go on the school camp or sleep over at friends. She feels that her friends might not want to see her, which further compounds her anxiety and low mood. It seems that Sara is experiencing the range and extent of worry which would indicate that she has generalized anxiety disorder (GAD) (Hudson et al. 2004).

2   What is generalized anxiety disorder (GAD)?

A Everyone has worries and feelings of anxiety as part of everyday life. Often this can serve a useful function; for example, if we need to sit an exam, a slight increase in our level of anxiety will make us more alert and vigilant and help us to perform better.

Generalized anxiety disorder (GAD) is a specific sub-type of anxiety where the person is constantly worried about a range of different issues beyond what might be regarded as normal. Table 4.1 shows the difference between normal worry and generalized anxiety disorder (GAD).

Table 4.1 Normal worry versus generalized anxiety disorder (GAD)

Normal worry	GAD
Worry does not prevent the carrying out of everyday tasks	Worrying disrupts schoolwork, leisure activities and social life
The worry can be controlled	Worry is uncontrollable
The worry, while uncomfortable, is not distressing	Worry is stressful and cannot be mitigated
Worry is limited to a narrow range of realistic concerns	Worry is about many things and tends to focus on the worst outcome
Worrying is brief or for a time-limited period	Worry occurs every day over a prolonged period

Anxiety has a number of physiological features. In Sara's case, these include:

- difficulty sleeping;
- poor concentration;
- difficulties with memory;
- rapid heartbeat;
- dizziness;
- rapid breathing;
- muscle tension;
- shaking from anxiety while waiting for the school bus;
- feeling a sense of constant nervous tension.

Often people also experience:

- the sensation of butterflies in the stomach;
- light-headedness, or difficulty breathing, for example, a choking feeling;
- the need to visit the toilet more frequently to pass urine or to have diarrhoea due to their anxiety;
- feeling excessively hot and sweaty.

The physical discomfort which occurs with anxiety often exacerbates the person's worry, which worsens the problem. The significant amount of energy, which the physiological features of anxiety use up, together with the fact that the person may already not sleep as well as they normally might, result in their mood becoming lower, as is the case with Sara.

The assessment proceeded with the CAMHS worker collecting Sara's family history, observing Sara's and Jan's interaction and speaking to each of them separately.

Family history

It is helpful to identify significant family members in order to understand the family composition. The CAMHS worker asked Sara with the help of her mum to construct a three-generational family tree, or genogram to which Sara added family names and ages (Eminson 2005).

The genogram was also used to explore the nature of the family relationships and to gather information on family health, patterns of coping, and resilience factors. Sara is an only child and described herself as shy, sensitive and inhibited, particularly in unfamiliar situations. It has been suggested that anxiety can occur through intergenerational transmission in the form of relationship patterns being repeated through learned behaviour and acquired coping responses (Barrett and Turner 2004). Sara's parents' own childhoods and experience of being parented are also directly connected to Sara's difficulties. For example, there is a history of anxiety in Simon's family. Simon's mother had panic disorder which led him to feel very protective towards his mother throughout his life. Three years ago he had to take six months off work with stress and panic for which he received cognitive behavioural therapy (CBT).

Jan experienced mild anxiety and depression after the sudden death of her father when she was 16, for which she received bereavement counselling. Jan describes a very close relationship to her own father, similar to that of Sara and Simon. Jan also later identified when speaking separately with the CAMHS worker that she had experienced **post-natal depression** following Sara's birth. Any family history of depression or bipolar disorder needs to be explored (NICE 2011), as evidence suggests that GAD in adolescence precedes the onset of major depression in adult life (Goodyer 2005).

Observation

Watching family interactions often provides insight into relationships. For example, difficulties in the **attachment** between a mother and younger child might be evident through a lack of physical contact, poor engagement and the mother not wanting to play with the child. The CAMHS worker observed Sara and Jan in the clinic waiting room and their interaction during the assessment.

In the waiting room Sara was huddled close to Jan, with her head down. Jan was affectionate towards Sara, and had her arm wrapped around her. During the assessment Sara resisted making eye contact, showed signs of anxiety by being restless, constantly picking at her jumper and distractedly fiddling with her bag when being asked questions. Jan tended to talk for Sara and provided more help to Sara than was needed and her desire to protect Sara from distress was clear.

At the mid-point during the assessment, Sara was seen separately, and asked questions concerning possible substance use or misuse, self-harm, **bullying** and safety issues. Protocols for safeguarding children would be followed if safety was a concern.

Jan was then seen separately and asked about any issues which might be better discussed without Sara being present. These included Jan's pregnancy with Sara and the post-birth period and relational aspects of her marriage with Simon (Eminson 2005). Jan experienced mild post-natal depression following Sara's birth but recognized the symptoms and received counselling and ongoing support from her health visitor. In the first year of life Sara had sleep difficulties and colic. Sara had mild separation anxiety on starting pre-school at the age of 3 but this resolved itself over the course of time. Children with anxiety disorders tend to have more difficulties adjusting to transitions (Rapee and Szollos 1997, cited in Hudson et al. 2004).

Communication between Sara's parents had deteriorated towards the end of their marriage with there being constant tension and disagreement and arguments. Jan was unclear as to the effect of this upon Sara who, whenever asked about how she felt regarding her parents' separating, seemed not to have an opinion.

3 **What screening and assessment tools should be used in assessing the severity of Sara's symptoms of GAD?**

A Before being referred to the CAMHS out-patient service Sara was screened using the Child Global Assessment Scale (CGAS). This is a key outcome measure and forms part of the National CAMHS Dataset.

CGAS is used by mental health clinicians to rate generally the everyday life functioning of children younger than 18 years of age. For a referral to the CAMHS specialist secondary services, a CGAS rating of 60 or less must be recorded. Sara scored 50, indicating a moderate degree of interference in functioning (the CGAS categories and scores can be found at: http://www.rcpsych.ac.uk/pdf).

At the assessment meeting, the severity of Sara's anxiety was measured using the Beck's Youth Inventory for both depression (BDI) and anxiety (BAI). Sara had an above average score for anxiety and a mildly impaired mood (Beck et al. 2005).

4 **What actions might be taken to help Sara?**

A Sara, like many children and young people, is receiving statutory education and is involved with both the school nurse and CAMHS. The CAMHS worker asked Sara's and Jan's permission to contact the school nurse and the school (Dogra and Baldwin 2009).

It has increasingly been highlighted that the multiple agencies which are involved with children and younger people need to effectively liaise and communicate in order to be of optimum effect for the child or young person. Among the advantages are:

- the effective coordination of care;
- the offer of multiple different professional perspectives and skill sets in the planning of care and allowing greater potential for the child's or young person's needs to be heard and understood;
- more opportunities to monitor the child or young person's mental state and progress.

However, in order to be effective, multi-agency input is required. Therefore, a meeting was arranged for Sara and Jan, Simon, the school nurse, Sara's teacher and the CAMHS worker to discuss how Sara might be supported and her mental health promoted. At the meeting, it was agreed that:

- Sara would feel more in control of her anxiety in the classroom by the use of a Cue card or Excuse me card which could be shown if she needed to leave the classroom.
- Sara would have regular one-to-one sessions with the CAMHS worker, where she was encouraged to express her views and feelings and address her anxiety and worries using a structured approach.
- Family work would be carried out by a family therapist with Sara and Jan on a fortnightly basis with Simon attending monthly.

• Even though they were separated Sara's parents agreed to receive **couple counselling** from a family therapist.

Sara found that knowing that she had the Cue card or Excuse me card gave her a great deal of reassurance and she did not need to use it. The sessions with the CAMHS helped Sara to work on her interpretation and understanding of what was happening around her. By talking about her greatest source of anxiety of her parents' separation Sara was able to challenge **catastrophic thoughts** such as: 'I cannot cope without my dad.' Sara instead challenged such thoughts and built more positive alternatives. For example, if something occurred which she thought her dad might like to know, she was encouraged to think: 'Next time I see my dad I will tell him that . . .'. The work with the school nurse also allowed Sara to reflect upon her relationship towards her parents and accept the changes which had occurred, so that while she no longer lived with her dad, she could still see him regularly.

The CAMHS worker explained to Sara how our thoughts affect our feelings and her catastrophic thinking had led to an escalation in her anxiety. Sara felt greatly empowered through this learning, and more in control of her thoughts and consequently the emotions which these triggered. She realized that she had become very self-focused and critical of herself and others and was also able to extend this new understanding to other areas of her life. Sara identified that thoughts such as: 'I don't think I can handle seeing my friends any more, I feel sick and scared' had eroded her confidence and led to her isolating herself, and continuing to think negatively and not being exposed to other sources of stimulation and ideas had reduced her confidence and lowered her mood. Also in relation to her schoolwork, Sara realized that thoughts such as: 'If I do my schoolwork, it will all go wrong' were self-defeating and had a harmful effect.

The **family-based work** involved the family therapist collaborating with Sara and Jan in fortnightly family meetings, but also with Simon attending monthly. This enabled them to find new ways of being together and relating to one another. The family therapist enhanced Sara's parents' knowledge and understanding of the physiological and psychological nature of Sara's anxiety, and how to help manage and prevent its reoccurrence. Both parents encouraged Sara to resume her interests and friendships. Even though their long-term plan was not to get back together, Jan and Simon received couple counselling from the family therapist in order to improve their relationship to help Sara.

Table 4.2 shows the therapeutic benefits of using both Sara's sessions with the school nurse, and family-based work for Sara.

CONCLUSION

Over time Sara's mood improved, she found it easier to sleep and began to resume many of the activities which she had stopped. Sara found that the techniques which she used in the sessions with the school nurse helped her with other problems and she gained in confidence. Sara feels that the added knowledge she has gained has improved her self-understanding and insight into how our thinking affects mood and feelings and that she is now able to manage her anxiety much better. Jan and Simon's relationship with each other and with Sara became better and Simon saw Sara more frequently.

Table 4.2 Therapeutic benefits for Sara and her parents

Sessions with the school nurse	Family-based work
Sara learned to identify physical symptoms accompanying the worry. She was taught deep breathing techniques and **progressive muscle relaxation** to control tension associated with anxiety. This consequently reduced the physical sensations of anxiety	Her parents were helped to find alternative ways of understanding and managing Sara's anxiety. Jan was discouraged from sitting for long periods with Sara at bedtimes and listening to her worries. Both parents helped Sara to use cognitive strategies such as relaxation techniques, thought stopping and distraction
Sara began to recognize the relationship between thoughts, feelings and behaviour. She learned to identify, challenge and change anxious thoughts, further reducing the physical sensations of anxiety	The therapy explored how the family were relating with each other since Simon left. The good aspects of home life prior to the family breakdown were identified which enabled everyone to value each other
Social problem solving helped to rebuild Sara's confidence in relating to friends and brought about behavioural change, i.e. positive self-talk and resuming interests and activities outside of the home environment	Couple counselling helped both Jan and Simon to address marital issues, conflicts, and ways of relating to each other with particular regard to Sara. A consistent parental approach was agreed upon. Sara's parents were able to achieve amicable relations with each other and consequently this helped Sara feel less burdened and more supported by her parents
Self-monitoring of progress enabled Sara to recognize how positive-thinking strategies could be successfully used in many situations. She was also able to predict future problems and knew how to manage these using her newly found coping skills	Simon agreed to provide a structure for consistent contact with Sara via telephone, Skype and visits, making expectations clear and providing stable conditions
Finally, work on separation from the therapist occurred	

REFERENCES

Barrett, P.M. and Turner, C.M. (2004) Prevention of childhood anxiety and depression, in P.M. Barrett and T.H. Ollendick (eds) *Handbook of Interventions that Work with Children and Adolescents: Prevention and Treatment*. Chichester: John Wiley & Sons, Ltd.

Beck, J.S., Beck, A.T., Jolly, J.B. and Steer, R.A (2005) *Beck Youth Inventories for Children and Adolescents Manual*, 2nd edn. San Antonio, TX: Pearson Education Inc.

Child Global Assessment Scale, available at: http://www.rcpsych.ac.uk/pdf/CGAS%20Ratings%20Guide.pdf (accessed 20 October 2011).

DoH (Department of Health) (2008) *Refocusing the Care Plan Approach: Policy and Positive Practice Guidance*. London: Department of Health.

Dogra, N. and Baldwin, L. (2009) Nursing assessment in CAMH, in N. Dogra and S. Leighton (eds) *Nursing in Child and Adolescent Mental Health.* Maidenhead: Open University Press.

Eminson, M. (2005) Assessment in child and adolescent psychiatry, in S.G. Gower (ed.) *Seminars in Child and Adolescent Psychiatry,* 2nd edn. London: Royal College of Psychiatrists.

Goodyer, I.M. (2005) Continuities and discontinuities from childhood to adult life, in S.G. Gower (ed.) *Seminars in Child and Adolescent Psychiatry,* 2nd edn. London: Royal College of Psychiatrists.

Hudson, J.L., Hughes, A.A. and Kendall, P.C. (2004) Treatment of generalized anxiety disorder in children and adolescents, in P.M. Barrett and T.H. Ollendick (eds) *Handbook of Interventions that Work with Children and Adolescents: Prevention and Treatment.* Chichester: John Wiley & Sons, Ltd.

Mattis, S.G. and Ollendick, T.H. (2002) *Panic Disorder and Anxiety in Adolescence.* PACTS 2. Oxford: BPS Blackwell.

NICE (National Institute of Health and Clinical Excellence) (2011) *Generalised Anxiety Disorder and Panic Disorder with or without Agoraphobia in Adults: Management in Primary and Secondary Community Care.* NICE Clinical Guideline 113. Available at: http://www.nice.org.uk/nicemedia/live/13314/52599/52599.pdf (accessed 23 October 2011).

CASE STUDY 5
Behaviour problems in children
Alison Coad

Joshua is 8 years old and lives with his mother Sarah, who is 30, and stepfather Rick, aged 38. He has a younger brother, Nathan, who is 6, and his mother is expecting a baby in four months time. Joshua's parents separated five years ago and he and his brother see his father regularly, spending every other weekend and some of the school holidays with him. Joshua gets on well with his stepfather.

Joshua has always been a lively child but recently his mother has noticed that he is becoming very rude, especially towards her. He refuses to tidy up his bedroom, and often has to be reminded to pick up his school bag and jacket which he drops in the hallway when he gets home. Joshua's mother is becoming exasperated with him and often threatens that she will take away treats – such as his games console – if he does not do as he is asked. However, she never follows through on this, as the one time that she did, Joshua made such a fuss that she ended up giving in to him half an hour later.

Nathan has started to pick up on Joshua's behaviour and is copying some of it. This has led to Sarah becoming anxious and irritable, and she has found that she spends a lot of time shouting at the boys. Last week she became so upset that she ended up shutting them in their room for an hour. Joshua spent this time drawing all over the bedroom walls with felt pen, encouraging Nathan to join in. The room had recently been decorated and for Sarah, this felt like 'the last straw'. When she attended her last ante-natal appointment, Sarah broke down in tears while describing the situation to the midwife.

1 **What issues should a healthcare professional consider in a situation such as this?**

A It is necessary to ascertain whether there is any risk of harm to a vulnerable individual. All NHS Trusts have policies for dealing with the protection of vulnerable children, adults and older persons; this is generally known as 'safeguarding' (Care Quality Commission 2010; see the Health and Social Care Act, 2008). When young children are involved, it is important for the healthcare professional to assess whether there are any indications that the child or children may be at risk of harm. Sarah's disclosure that she 'shut the children in their room for an hour' would need to be discussed in more detail, and considered in context.

Areas to explore would be what the children have access to while in the room (any potential dangers such as open windows or hot radiators); whether the children were locked in the room, or whether the door was just closed; and how distressing the children found the experience. If a professional has any concerns about these or any other issues that would suggest that Sarah's actions were abusive or neglectful, then they have a duty of care to refer those concerns to an agency such as Children's Services, who have procedures in place to investigate and, if necessary, act on these concerns.

Having spent some time talking with Sarah, the midwife is satisfied that the events that Sarah described were a one-off episode precipitated by a build-up of stress over recent months. There is nothing to suggest that Joshua and Nathan have been harmed by their experience, or that it is a regular occurrence. The midwife advises Sarah to make an appointment with her G P to see if there might be any additional support that Sarah could be offered.

The G P has known Sarah and her family since the birth of the children and is concerned to hear about her difficulties with Joshua's behaviour. Sarah suffered post-natal depression after Nathan's birth which required treatment with anti-depressant medication. She asks Sarah to complete a questionnaire (the **PHQ-9**) to see whether or not Sarah might be suffering from symptoms of depression. The score shows no indication of clinical depression, but Sarah admits that she has been feeling very upset about the boys and that she is particularly worried about how she will manage when the new baby arrives.

2   **What services might be available to support Sarah?**

A   In the first instance, Sarah's G P could seek advice from a CAMHS primary mental health worker.

3   **What is the role of the primary mental health worker?**

A   Primary mental health worker, or P M H W, was a role established following recommendations in a report published by the N H S Health Advisory Service in 1995. Their role is to act as a specialist liaison service between primary care professionals, such as G Ps and school nurses, and the local Child and Adolescent Mental Health Services (CAMHS). The service has expanded over recent years (Hickey et al. 2007, cited in Richardson et al. 2010).

With Sarah's permission, the G P contacts the surgery's P M H W and discusses Sarah's case. The P M H W suggests that it would be useful for a CAMHS worker to undertake an initial assessment, as the difficulties have been developing over several months and the G P is concerned about Sarah's mental health. Although Sarah is not depressed, she is clearly distressed and the G P is concerned that she may be susceptible to another episode of post-natal depression if she does not receive support at this stage.

A CAMHS worker, Jane, offers Sarah an initial appointment. She agrees to visit Sarah and the boys at home to undertake an assessment of the current situation. Jane asks to speak with Sarah on her own in the first instance.

4   **What is the rationale for talking to Sarah without her children if the main problem seems to be the children's behaviour?**

A   It is important for Jane to be able to gain a clear picture of Sarah's concerns, and it is likely that this will entail detailed descriptions of problem behaviour. Jane does not want the children to have to listen to an account that may make them feel embarrassed or defensive. She also needs an honest and open account and Sarah may be inhibited if the children are present. However, it is equally important to involve the children directly at some point in the assessment to ensure that their needs and wishes are acknowledged within any treatment plan that is devised (Helm 2010).

Jane talks with Sarah about the family history and learns that Joshua's behaviour has become more challenging over the past six months. Prior to this, Sarah had not had any significant concerns, although she admits that she has found it difficult to work out how to discipline the boys since Rick moved into the family home. Rick does not have any children of his own and Sarah explains that he does not feel that it is his role to discipline the boys.

When Sarah lived with the boys' father, she found it easier to manage because he tended to be the one who made the rules. The boys would listen to him, and this is still the case, as recently Sarah has had a conversation with him and he is not experiencing any problems with the boys when they stay with him. Since Sarah became pregnant, she has been feeling increasingly tired and has found that she has less time to spend with the boys. She also admits that she tends to 'turn a blind eye' to things that she would not have allowed in the past – for example, if the children refuse to go to bed when she tells them to, she no longer insists and allows them to stay up later.

Joshua and Nathan are both doing well at school and there have been no reports of behaviour problems from teachers.

Jane spends some time talking with the boys as part of the assessment.

5　**What issues would Jane need to think about when she meets Joshua and Nathan?**

A　The primary level of assessment would focus on whether the boys' basic needs are being met – are they clean, appropriately clothed, and well nourished? Are their emotional needs met within their home environment? Assuming that there are no obvious concerns with respect to these areas, Jane would need to assess whether the boys are within normal range for physical growth and emotional and intellectual development. These developmental stages are sometimes referred to as 'milestones'. At the age of 8, a child is likely to be becoming more independent and will therefore need clear guidance from his or her parents on rules and boundaries within and outside the home. A child of 6, particularly a child with an older sibling, is also likely to demonstrate more independent behaviour, for example, in their self-care and social interactions.

Jane would also need to evaluate Joshua's and Nathan's behaviour in the context of Sarah's concerns. As a **CAMHS Tier 2** worker, she would be alert to the possibility of the difficulties that Sarah has described being symptomatic of more pervasive problems such as **conduct disorder** or **oppositional defiant disorder**, an anxiety disorder, or depression. Difficulties of this nature are likely to require intervention by **CAMHS Tier 3** professionals, and may include an assessment by a psychiatrist.

Joshua and Nathan are happy to meet Jane and they appear to enjoy chatting with her. Joshua is keen to tell Jane about his football team and his best friend at school. Nathan is shy, but is happy to sit and draw while Jane talks to Joshua. When Jane asks the boys about rules at home, and who makes them, Joshua laughs and says that: 'Nobody makes rules here except me. I can do what I like here.' He admits that he acts differently when he is at his father's house, and that he 'listens to what dad says because if I didn't I'd get into trouble'. Jane notices that Sarah has tears in her eyes when Joshua says this.

6　**Based on the information gathered by Jane during her assessment, does Sarah's family need any intervention from mental health professionals?**

A　Jane takes the results of her assessment back to her team to discuss her impressions and to suggest that Sarah and Rick might benefit from some support around their parenting. There is no evidence of any developmental problem for either of the boys, and their behaviour in other environments, for example, at their father's house and at school does not present any problems. The key issue appears to be the fact that Joshua and Nathan are unclear about rules and boundaries when they are at home with Sarah and Rick. Sarah feels that she has to manage a lot of the difficult aspects of parenting without Rick's support, as he is unsure what his role is. She has lost confidence in her ability to make decisions about the behaviour of her children and has therefore become inconsistent in the messages that she gives them.

The team agreed that a referral to the CAMHS service parenting group would be appropriate which involves attendance at 12 weekly sessions. Jane contacted Sarah to discuss the possibility of referring her and Rick to the parenting group.

Sarah is not keen to attend as she is not sure how it could make a difference to Joshua's behaviour. After some discussion, Jane realizes that Sarah is very anxious at the prospect of having to attend a group because she is worried that she will be embarrassed by having to share her problems with strangers. She also admits that she feels judged by the CAMHS team. She sees the referral to the parenting group as meaning that her parenting is not good enough.

Jane offers Sarah reassurance by telling her that many parents experience worries and problems that are significant enough for them to seek outside help. The evidence for this is that the group is run three times each year and is always full. The group leaders get lots of positive feedback from parents and most parents who enrol complete the course. Sarah agrees to try the group but is still unsure about exactly what will be involved.

7 **What evidence is there to support the use of parenting groups?**

A Parenting groups, sometimes referred to as parent training programmes, have been the subject of a great deal of research which has shown an impressive success rate (Cartwright-Hatton et al. 2010). The best known of these courses are The Incredible Years Programme and Triple P. Further information about these programmes is available via the websites listed in the further reading.

8 **What would a parenting group involve?**

A Parenting groups aim to provide skills training for parents who are struggling to manage the behaviour of their children. Cartwright-Hatton et al. (2010: 8) observe that:

> Standard programmes (i.e. the ones developed for children with behavioural problems) are based on strong evidence that such children have parents who employ a number of behaviours that are thought to cause, or at least maintain, their child's difficulties. It is these parenting behaviours that the intervention seeks to modify.

It is essential for this message to be conveyed in a sensitive manner, as many parents like Sarah express anxieties. Emphasizing existing strengths and skills, as well as the highly demanding nature of parenting, can help to reassure parents. Part of the benefit of the group format is the opportunity it provides for parents to meet and gain support from others in similar situations.

The key principles of Webster-Stratton's 1994 approach involve strengthening the relationship between the parent and child prior to helping the parent to develop strategies to manage difficult behaviour (Webster-Stratton and Herbert 1994). Early sessions focus on the importance of play and praise, developing communication skills and problem-solving. Towards the end of the programme, techniques such as boundary-setting, establishing clear household rules, and ways of managing undesirable behaviours are introduced. The programme is usually run over a period of 12 weeks, and parents are asked to attend without their children.

By the time of their next appointment, Sarah had attended the first three sessions of the parenting group and has already made some changes. She told Jane that she had not realized how little time she had been spending with her sons lately. Each session of the group sets the parents tasks to carry out at home. The first of these tasks was to spend more time playing with the children, and Sarah has been setting aside half an hour each afternoon to do this. Joshua and Nathan are both excited about this, and Sarah has noticed that Joshua is more relaxed after they have spent some time together doing an activity of his choice.

Sarah has also made an effort to notice when the children do something helpful – she has set up a rewards system which involves putting a marble into a jam jar every time they help with a household chore, or put their toys away without having to be reminded. The family sat down together and worked out what tasks would earn a marble. The results are written on a list stuck to the kitchen cupboard. When the jar is full, the children are allowed to choose a treat from a list that includes a comic, going to the cinema, or staying up for an extra half an hour. Marbles are only ever earned and never taken away. This way the children feel motivated to behave well and emphasis is placed on positive behaviours rather than negative.

Although there have still been incidents when Joshua has been rude or has refused to do as he is asked, Sarah and Rick have agreed that they will ignore the bad behaviour if possible. They have also worked out a strategy between them to ensure that they are both giving the children the same messages – one of the problems they had in the past was that if Sarah said no to something, Joshua would go and ask Rick, who tended to say yes. Sarah has also had a conversation with her former husband, who is very supportive and who has agreed on fixed rules such as bedtime and how much time Joshua is allowed to play on the computer.

Jane offers Sarah a follow-up appointment in 6 months' time. Sarah and Rick completed the parenting group and they have introduced some important changes to their routines at home. Joshua is still prone to answer back and has occasionally had tantrums where he has broken things in his room. However, with the help of the parenting group tutors and fellow parents at the group, Sarah and Rick have devised some clear rules about the consequences of Joshua's difficult behaviour. These rules include sanctions such as the loss of ten minutes' computer time if he is rude to another member of the family. Sarah admits that she still finds it difficult to stick to this at times, but that with Rick backing her up, it has become a lot easier to manage. The new baby has arrived in the household without any major upsets.

Jane provides Sarah and Rick with details of websites where they can access ongoing help and advice should they feel the need for some extra help in the future, for example, http://www.familylives.org.uk, which offers a 24-hour confidential helpline, and Relate, which provides advice on all aspects of family relationships. They are aware that if new or more complex problems emerge in the future, they can seek a re-referral to CAMHS via their GP.

REFERENCES

Care Quality Commission (2010) *Protocol on Safeguarding*. Available at: http://www.cqc.org.uk/_db/_documents/20100607_Final_Final_Comms_edit_protocol_final_additions_201008181151_201010015932.doc (accessed 30 July 2011).

Cartwright-Hatton, S., Laskey, B., Rust, S. and McNally, D. (2010) *From Timid to Tiger: A Treatment Manual for Parenting the Anxious Child*. Chichester: Wiley-Blackwell.

Helm, D. (2010) *Making Sense of Child and Family Assessment: How to Interpret Children's Needs*. London: Jessica Kingsley.

Richardson, G., Partridge, I. and Barrett, J. (2010) *Child and Adolescent Mental Health Services: An Operational Handbook.* 2nd edn. London: RC Psych Publications.

Richardson, G. and Wyatt, A. (2010) CAMHS in context, in G. Richardson, I. Partridge, and J. Barrett (eds) *Child and Adolescent Mental Health Services: An Operational Handbook.* 2nd edn. London: RC Psych Publications.

Webster-Stratton, C. and Herbert, M. (1994) *Troubled Families – Problem Children. Working with Families: A Collaborative Process.* Chichester: John Wiley & Sons, Ltd.

FURTHER READING

American Psychiatric Association (2000) *Diagnostic and Statistical Manual of Mental Disorders,* 4th edn (text revision). Washington, DC: APA.

NHS Health Advisory Service (1995) *Together We Stand: Commissioning, Role and Management of Child and Adolescent Mental Health Services.* London: HMSO.

Relate. Available at: http://www.relateforparents.org.uk (accessed 31 July 2011).

Role of primary care mental health worker. Available at: http://www.cypnow.co.uk/Careers/article/1063510/Careers-CAMHS-primary-mental-health-worker/ (accessed 30 July 2011).

Royal College of Psychiatrists (2004) *Factsheet: Behavioural and Conduct Problems; and Good Parenting.* Available at: http://www.rcpsych.ac.uk/mentalhealthinformation/childrenandyoungpeople.aspx (accessed 31 July 2011).

Slater, A. and Bremner, G. (eds) (2003) *An Introduction to Developmental Psychology.* Oxford: Blackwell Publishing.

The Incredible Years. Available at: http://www.incredibleyears.com (accessed 31 July 2011).

The Triple P (Positive Parenting Programme). Available at: http://www.triplep.net/ (accessed 1 August 2011).

Whittington, C.J., Kendall, T., Fonagy, P., Cottrell, D., Cotgrove, A. and Boddington, E. (2004) Selective serotonin reuptake inhibitors in childhood depression: systematic review of published versus unpublished data, *The Lancet,* 363(9418): 1341–5.

Sally and John have two children – Ellie, aged 12, and Daniel, aged 16. They separated three years ago and since then John has met a new partner, Rachel, who also has two children, and he recently moved into her house. John's parents live locally and he is close to them.

Sally's mother died when she was a teenager and she does not see her father very often. Since the separation, Sally has felt isolated from John's parents, feeling that they blame her for the marriage breakdown. Sally has recently been diagnosed with clinical depression, and she has been prescribed anti-depressants by her GP.

Daniel is getting on well at school and does not appear to be struggling too much with the recent changes in his family. He has a wide group of friends and is very involved in a drama group, which means he is often out in the evenings and at weekends. Daniel still gets on well with his father, and sees him regularly.

Ellie was very upset by her father's new relationship and has not been able to build a relationship with Rachel. She has refused to visit John in his new home, and has told her mum that she believes that: 'Dad loves his new family more than us.' Ellie has started to stay out late and has been getting into trouble at school. Unknown to her parents, Ellie has been smoking and drinking. Two weeks ago Ellie stole a number of her mother's tablets and took an overdose of fluoxetine and paracetamol. After she took the tablets, she became frightened and told her mother who took her to the Accident and Emergency department at the local hospital.

1 **What are the key issues to consider at an initial assessment of a young person who has self-harmed?**

A The most important factor is the risk of Ellie's propensity for further self-harm. The fact that Ellie told her mother about the overdose very soon after it happened, and also that she took relatively few tablets suggest that Ellie's actions were impulsive and that she had not thought about the consequences of her actions. However, each case needs to be approached as a new situation and a thorough assessment of Ellie's understanding of the potential effects of the overdose and overall mental state is necessary.

When the nurse in Accident and Emergency questioned Ellie about the overdose, it emerged that Ellie believed that the number of tablets that she took could kill her. She told the nurse that at the time of taking the tablets she wanted to die because she felt that her life was 'such a mess'. She had not planned the overdose in advance, but had taken the tablets following a particularly bad day at school and an argument with her father about not wanting to visit him. Ellie denied any other form of self-harm prior to this incident, but said that there had been times when she felt as though she no longer wanted to live. Ellie also admitted getting drunk on two or three occasions, once to the point where she could not remember everything she had done.

2 **What other kinds of behaviour, apart from an overdose, might be considered as self-harm?**

A As part of a thorough risk assessment, it is important to ask questions about a range of behaviours. These include:

- deliberate self-harm by cutting;
- consumption of excessive amounts of alcohol;
- use of illicit substances such as street drugs;
- risky behaviours such as unprotected sexual activity.

Risk assessment also needs to cover whether the client is at risk from others, or might be at risk of causing harm to others.

Once it was agreed that Ellie was medically fit to leave the hospital, her doctor agreed to allow her to go home but referred her for an urgent appointment at the local Child and Adolescent Mental Health Services. Ellie was given an appointment at the Child and Adolescent clinic the following day.

At this appointment, Ellie and her mum saw a nurse therapist who undertook an initial assessment.

3 **What other issues, apart from risk, might an initial assessment of Ellie include?**

A When undertaking any mental health assessment, it is important to understand the context within which problems might have developed. This is particularly important when working with children and adolescents such as Ellie, as factors such as family difficulties, problems at school, or peer pressure can have a huge impact on the young person's well-being. Variables such as the young person's developmental stage, social circumstances, educational ability and individual disposition will all influence the way in which a young person responds to difficulties.

Typical issues covered within an initial assessment of a young person such as Ellie might therefore include:

- family history (including medical and psychiatric history);
- developmental history of the young person;
- family structure – whether the young person lives with their parents, or, as in Ellie's case, there are other arrangements;
- which family members are most important to the young person;
- how the young person perceives the current situation, and what they consider to be the problems;
- the onset and duration of the current difficulties;
- what kind of help, if any, the young person would like to receive;
- an initial formulation of the young person's difficulties, which might include a diagnosis and suggested treatment strategies.

The nurse therapist identifies that Ellie's current difficulties stem from the breakdown of her parents' marriage, and her relationship with her father and his new partner. These issues have led to symptoms of depression and to problems at school. The therapist suggests an appointment with the clinic's systemic therapist.

4 **What are the key features of a systemic approach?**

A Systemic therapy examines the different environments and influences that combine to make up every person's life. For Ellie, the systems that create her world are those of her family, her school life, her **peer group** and broader cultural categories such as class, gender and race. If problems arise, the systemic approach would look to the causes and effects of these problems within the system as a whole. Individual psychopathology is regarded as a part of a bigger picture that includes family and social contexts.

Professionals who are called upon to assist a family are a part of the social context and are therefore not seen as 'experts' who know how to fix the family's problems. Instead, family and professionals become part of the same team, with the aim of problem-solving together.

5 **Why might systemic therapy be an appropriate intervention for Ellie and her family?**

A The fact that Ellie has taken an overdose might be seen as a symptom of depression, but the cause of her depression can be recognized as arising from the effects of disruption to her key caring relationships. Her father's new relationship has created a rift in Ellie's relationship with him, as she feels he is no longer available to her. She does not know how to express this, but she does know that it makes her feel sad, angry and rejected.

Ellie's father was brought up in a strongly **patriarchal** family where children were expected to unquestioningly obey their parents' wishes and be obedient. As he has never had reason to question that model, he finds it difficult to recognize that Ellie might need to express her grief at the loss of her family life. Ellie's mother has become depressed herself and is therefore less able to offer emotional support to Ellie.

Ellie's brother Daniel is able to create new relationships outside the family, and so feels less threatened by his parents' separation and his father's new relationship and is less in need of them than Ellie. The succession of losses and shifts within the family's relationships has left Ellie feeling confused and uncertain. Ellie has experienced low mood which has affected her performance at school and her relationship with friends. The changes in one system (Ellie's family) have therefore impacted on other systems (school, peer group) and have led Ellie to experiment with behaviours that challenge the expectations of her family and her cultural group.

On receiving notification of an appointment with the systemic therapist, Ellie is uncertain about what will happen, and fearful that they will: 'tell her off'. Sally feels responsible for the problems that have occurred, and is worried that the therapist will think that she is a bad mother. Neither Ellie nor Sally feel able to express these worries, but on meeting them it is clear to the therapist that they are both anxious.

6 **How would the systemic therapist begin the conversation with Sally and Ellie? What would the therapist want to achieve in the first session?**

A The most important aspect of an initial meeting is to engage the clients in the process and to build a rapport with them. The therapist can do this in a range of ways – for example, warm and friendly demeanour, clear explanations of what will happen in the appointment, and information about the way that systemic therapy can be helpful. It is important that the family feel that they are an active part of the process and that they have control over how the session is conducted.

Systemic therapy looks at the relationships between members of a system and encourages members of the system to understand how life might be feeling for others by putting themselves in their shoes. It is therefore very important that the therapist is able to understand the way that the family communicates. This process is similar to learning a new language, in order to ensure that the family can tell their story in a way that is meaningful to them, which White and Epston (1990) describe as **narrative therapy** or storytelling.

It is also important to understand the structure of the family from Ellie and Sally's perspective by establishing who is important to whom and identifying family alliances and rifts. Diagrams can be very helpful to explore these questions – and constructing a genogram in the session, with the family's help is a useful exercise (Figure 6.1 shows Ellie and Sally's genogram, including their understanding of how family members get on together).

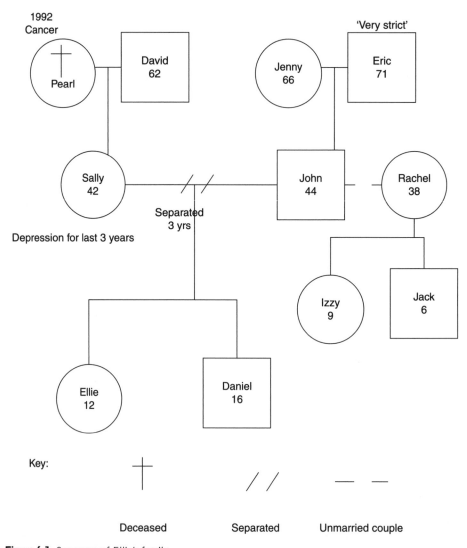

Figure 6.1 Genogram of Ellie's family

7 **What might the plan for future sessions be?**

A During the first session, when asked what they might like to change, Ellie and Sally spent much time describing interactions between Ellie and her father. The systemic therapist points this out and wonders if Ellie and Sally could invite Ellie's father to attend future sessions. Ellie is hesitant but says she would agree to this if her brother Daniel could also be invited, as she feels that Daniel has a good understanding of her relationship with her father.

The plan for the second session was therefore agreed. The systemic therapist explains that she and her colleague would work together with the family to gain a clear understanding of the situation. She explained that there are a range of approaches used within systemic therapy. These range from prescriptive approaches where the therapist can set tasks for the family to undertake between sessions (Palazzoli et al. 1978) to techniques involving the family in creative approaches, such as the multi-family therapy (MFT) approach proposed by Asen and Scholz (2010). MFT was developed in the 1940s and 1950s in the United States, and first applied in the UK in the 1970s. It is a dynamic approach requiring flexibility, curiosity and a willingness to experiment, both on the part of therapists and the families involved. Rudi Dallos (Dallos and Draper 2010) captures a sense of the process of MFT when he notes that: 'Multi-family therapy ... sessions have a feel of being at the circus, the theatre, stand-up comedy, children's party. Above all, they transform problems by fun, creativity and humour.'

Systemic therapy is often delivered by more than one therapist, in order to provide multiple perspectives and generate a range of hypotheses about the situation. The team can vary in size from two therapists to a large team of a dozen or more, although this is only really feasible if the clinic has a one-way mirror and observation room facility. This facility enables some members of the team to sit behind a one-way mirror and observe the therapy session, which is known as a reflecting team (Andersen 1987). Therapists in the team behind the screen can join the session at appropriate points to pose questions, ask for further information about particular issues, or to offer compliments or observations about the way that the family are responding to the process.

From agreement with Ellie and Sally in the first meeting with the systemic therapist it was decided to invite John and Daniel to subsequent sessions, while the systemic therapist invited a colleague to attend. However, the family declined the intervention of the full systemic team, as they did not feel comfortable with the idea of being observed from behind the screen.

At the next session, the family, the systemic therapist and her colleague started work with Ellie and Sally on constructing a diagram of the family dynamics. The therapists invited the family to think about a number of ways the family functioned. These included how each family member viewed the others, whether there was a hierarchy, the mutual influence of the individuals within the unit, and the relationships between them.

It was suggested that the family create a **family sculpting** which can be achieved by a variety of different methods, for example, using lengths of coloured rope to represent alliances and demarcations between family members. However, the approach which particularly appealed to Ellie, and, which was suggested by Asen and Scholz (2010), is clay modelling to create a three-dimensional representation of the family.

Ellie created a scenario with herself as a small figure outside the main family structure with John, Sally and Daniel as larger, more clearly defined figures forming a strong unit without her. None of the other family members represented themselves in this way, although Daniel's model depicted his father as a larger, stronger figure than the others.

This exercise provided an opportunity to discuss Ellie's feelings about her place in the family. Daniel was shocked to learn that Ellie felt so alone, and Sally and John were saddened to learn that their daughter felt so isolated.

The therapists worked with the family to devise some activities to carry out before the next session to help Ellie feel more a part of the family. It was agreed that John would spend some time with Ellie and Daniel, meeting for supper at a restaurant, agreeing that they would use this time to plan ways that they can meet together regularly. Sally acknowledged that her own low mood had made her less accessible and reluctant to relate to Ellie, and she agreed to seek individual counselling.

The systemic therapists offered six sessions and by the end of these Ellie had a regular arrangement in place to meet with her father at a neutral location away from his new home as she did not want to visit him at home at this stage but agrees that she will think about it in the future. Daniel offered to accompany Ellie on a visit to their father's new home when she feels ready. Ellie was also more settled at school, while Sally was offered counselling through her GP, and is more optimistic about her future.

REFERENCES

Andersen, T. (1987) The reflecting team: dialogue and meta-dialogue in clinical work, *Family Process*, 26: 415–28.

Asen, E. and Scholz, M. (2010) *Multi-Family Therapy: Concepts and Techniques*. Hove: Routledge.

Palazzoli, M.S., Boscolo, L., Cecchin, G. and Prata, G. (1978) A ritualized prescription in family therapy: odd days and even days, *Journal of Marital and Family Therapy*, 4(3): 3–9.

White, M. and Epston, D. (1990) *Narrative Means to Therapeutic Ends*. New York: WW Norton.

FURTHER READING

AFT (2009) *Summary of Family Interventions Recommended and Reviewed in NICE Guidelines*. Association for Family Therapy and Systemic Practice in the UK. Available at: www.aft.org.uk (accessed 29 May 2011).

Asen, E. (2004) Collaborating in promiscuous swamps: the systemic practitioner as context chameleon, *Journal of Family Therapy*, 26: 280–5.

Carr, A. (2006) *Family Therapy: Concepts Process and Practice*. Chichester: John Wiley & Sons, Ltd.

Carter, B. and McGoldrick, M. (eds) (1998) *The Expanded Family Life Cycle: Individual, Family and Social Perspectives*. Boston: Allyn and Bacon.

Cecchin, G. (1987) Hypothesizing, circularity, and neutrality revisited: an invitation to curiosity, *Family Process*, 26: 405–13.

Dallos, R. and Draper, R. (2010) *An Introduction to Family Therapy and Systemic Practice*, 3rd edn. Maidenhead: McGraw-Hill.

George, E., Iveson, C. and Ratner, H. (2000) *Problem to Solutions: Brief Therapy with Individuals and Families*, 2nd edn. London: BT Press.

NICE (National Institute for Health and Clinical Excellence) (2009) *Depression in Adults*. Clinical Guideline CG90. (Update). Available at: http: www.//guidance.nice.org.uk/CG90(accessed 13 March 2012).

Rivett, M. and Street, E. (2010) *Family Therapy: 100 Key Points and Techniques*. London: Routledge.

Simon, R.M. (1972) Sculpting the family, *Family Process*, 11: 49–57.

PART 2
Common Mental Health Problems in Adults

Generalized anxiety disorder (GAD)
Nick Wrycraft

Angela is 28 years old, and lives with her partner and their 2-year-old daughter and works part-time as a teaching assistant at a local primary school. Her partner recently lost his job and has since struggled to find work. Although she usually enjoys good health and rarely goes to the doctor, Angela has visited the GP a number of times over the past eight months and five times over the last three months with recurrent physical health issues. These include a number of stomach upsets, muscular tensions, back pain, minor breathlessness and difficulty sleeping.

During these appointments Angela has alluded to concerns and worries, but on her most recent visit she became very tearful and agitated, stating that she is still experiencing difficulty sleeping, feels overwhelmed with worries and is exhausted. While talking with the GP, Angela appeared to be restless, wringing her hands, clenching her jaw and rapidly tapping her foot.

When asked what her worries were, Angela said that she is concerned about coping financially due to her partner's employment difficulties, and that this has placed more pressure on her to provide for the family. Angela stated that recently due to being tired and anxious, she made an uncharacteristic mistake at work and is worried that she will make further errors with the consequence that she might lose her job and her financial situation worsen. She also feels guilty that her child attends nursery while she is at work and that she ought to be a 'better mother'. Angela admitted that she has felt low in mood and anxious for most of the past eight months. She says that she knows she is 'a worrier' and generally manages these feelings by keeping active.

The GP asked whether Angela feels that she is experiencing anxiety. Angela was initially surprised at the GP's comments as she had not thought that she was experiencing a mental health problem, however, several times recently she has felt as though she were 'going mad' due to how she was feeling. The GP suggested that Angela might benefit from taking anti-depressant medication. However, Angela was reluctant to go on medication but did agree to be assessed by a community psychiatric nurse (CPN) who liaises with the surgery. Angela reluctantly agreed, but was unsure how this might help.

1 **What are the physical and psychological features of anxiety?**

A Anxiety has a wide range of physical and psychological features. These include:

Physical symptoms

- restlessness;
- perspiring;
- **palpitations** or rapid heartbeat;

- feeling dizzy or faint;
- sensitivity to noise;
- feeling nauseous;
- shortness of breath, or choking;
- uneasiness or 'butterflies' in the stomach;
- needing to urinate frequently;
- diarrhoea or stomach upset;
- difficulty sleeping;
- muscular tension in the body.

Psychological symptoms

- feeling restless;
- experiencing events as happening very quickly;
- inability to concentrate or focus, for example, difficulty reading information;
- **hypervigilant**, or preoccupied with something which other people might regard as unimportant;
- feeling panicky;
- mental fatigue and tiredness;
- feeling anxious or afraid;
- feeling helpless and unable to influence events;
- feeling out of control, or as though 'I am going mad' or unusually irritable or angry;
- feeling tearful or upset;
- emotionally **labile** (changeable).

2   **What is generalized anxiety disorder (GAD)?**

A   Generalized anxiety disorder (GAD) is one of a range of mental health problems linked to anxiety. These include **acute stress disorder,** obsessive compulsive disorder (OCD), **panic,** phobia, and post-traumatic stress disorder (PTSD). All of these mental health problems have elements of anxiety but have distinctly different features and levels of severity (NCCMH 2011). The person with GAD may have some of the physical and psychological features identified above. However, GAD may be present when:

- The person worries uncontrollably nearly every day for six months.
- These worries are often experienced as intrusive thoughts or preoccupations.
- The focus shifts, so that the person worries about a range of different situations or issues.
- The worry is excessive in relation to the event or circumstance.
- The feelings are distressing for the person.
- The person's ability to function in everyday life and work is affected.

(NCCMH 2011; NHS Choices 2011)

Often GAD occurs co-morbidly with other physical and mental health problems and frequently depression, and is believed to affect around 1 in 20 people in the UK and more women than men (McManus et al. 2009; NCCMH 2011).

3 **Which aspects of GAD can you identify from the above outline of Angela's case?**

A Although there may be other explanations for these symptoms, over recent months Angela has had a number of physical features of anxiety, including stomach upsets, muscular tensions, back pain, minor breathlessness and difficulty sleeping. In the appointment with the GP Angela was also tearful and agitated and said she was exhausted, which might indicate physical and psychological fatigue as a result of anxiety. She also appeared to be anxious and was restless, wringing her hands, clenching her jaw and rapidly tapping her foot. Angela has had worries for over six months and in the discussion with the GP identified that she felt anxiety with regard to several situations or circumstances, and this might be considered excessive, which is consistent with GAD. Angela is also finding these worries distressing and due to her anxiety has made an uncharacteristic mistake at work suggesting that this is impacting upon her general capacity to function in everyday life. Angela also said she felt as though she is: 'going mad' which is a feeling occurring as a result of a loss of control and of events happening quickly.

In spite of being a frequently occurring health problem, GAD is often under-recognized within primary care settings. Some common reasons for this are present in Angela's case where her physical features have been treated as individual unconnected problems and the person might dismiss or underestimate that the multiple worries which they are feeling are due to anxiety.

4 **What causes GAD?**

A The cause of GAD is not known but in many cases it is thought to be due to a combination of factors:

- *biological processes* – anxiety is triggered by an imbalance in neurotransmitters, especially serotonin and noradrenaline, which can predispose the person to experience GAD or anxiety-related disorders.
- *genetic* – although no clear link has been made to suggest that members of the same family will experience GAD, there is a high incidence of members of families experiencing anxiety disorders (NCCMH 2011).
- *environment* – often living in poor environments, lack of education and employment and role within society.
- *experiences of traumatic events and abuse, poor parenting and having parents who are experiencing mental health problems* – all have the potential to predispose people to experiencing GAD. Conversely, good and supportive parenting has been identified as a protective mechanism against developing GAD (NCCMH 2011).
- *personality traits* – in some cases, people with GAD have personality traits whereby they are prone to anxiety, as is the case with Angela who describes herself as a 'worrier'. People with a propensity to worry can in some cases develop coping mechanisms which prove to be unsuccessful. Or alternatively, when confronted with challenging life events, find their capacity to cope is compromised.

Other causes of generalized anxiety disorder also include:

- drinking too much caffeine in tea or coffee;
- the side effects of some anti-depressant medication;
- an over-active thyroid, and the excessive release of the hormone thyroxine;
- illegal drugs;

- other physical health conditions, for example, **arrhythmia** (irregular heartbeat) which can cause anxiety;
- low blood sugar levels through not eating regularly (**hypoglycaemia**).

(Patient.co.uk 2011)

5   **What interventions might be helpful for Angela?**

A   Often GAD is experienced as an ongoing and recurrent problem, and early identification is important in ensuring that effective treatment can be accessed. Guidance suggests that treatment for GAD proceeds on a **stepped care** approach, with the least intensive intervention chosen (NCCMH 2011). Yet it is still important to work collaboratively and agree a treatment option which the person prefers. Among the range of interventions are individual therapy and groupwork.

INDIVIDUAL THERAPY

- Cognitive behavioural therapy (CBT) is a structured psychological approach in which the person works with the healthcare practitioner to identify the effects of their thoughts, beliefs and understanding on feelings, emotions and mental health. Through working with the healthcare practitioner the person can acquire and develop practical skills, techniques and coping resources to improve their mental health. The relationship is of time-limited duration with the purpose of empowering the person to take control of their life and identify proactive solutions to their problems.
- Counselling involves the person attending individual sessions with a therapist. While counselling approaches are varied and generic, often it takes the form of working towards agreed and negotiated goals.
- Signposting – increasingly, there has been an emphasis on making therapeutic resources available through the growing variety of communication media and technology. This serves to empower people by making help more easily and readily accessible without having to attend appointments or become involved on an ongoing basis with specialist mental health services. Often health care practitioners can direct people towards appropriate and evidence-based information on helpful therapeutic techniques such as relaxation and managing anxiety. The forms this information takes include:
  - leaflets
  - books
  - DVDs
  - tapes
  - downloads
  - **computerized CBT (CCBT)**
  - telephone support from healthcare professionals

GROUPWORK

- Groupwork with other people experiencing anxiety in the form of attending self-help groups, either through referral by healthcare professionals to day services or independent

agencies. Themed groups and programmes focus on a range of issues including **problem-solving**, assertiveness training, and relaxation, and run for a number of sessions.
* The person and their family or friends carrying out independent research, for example, on the internet where a wide range of useful sources of information is available, or at local library services which often stock user-friendly literature on common mental health problems.
* Medication – a range of medications have been identified as being effective in reducing anxiety, including some anti-depressants such as Selective Serotonin Reuptake Inhibitors (SSRIs) (Patient.co.uk 2011). However, these need to be taken in strict accordance with medical advice, and care taken to be vigilant for any side effects.

Often treatment will involve a combination of the above approaches depending on the person's preference and situation, as everyone will experience GAD differently.

ASSESSMENT

When meeting for an assessment with the CPN Angela was initially reluctant to engage. She felt that seeing a mental health professional reinforced her perception that she was not coping, which further undermined her confidence and self-esteem. The CPN was perceptive to Angela's concerns, and reassured her that many people have similar experiences of GAD. They also conducted the assessment in an informal and friendly manner while still acting professionally, and, although identifying her needs, also focused on her positive coping in spite of difficulties.

An assessment is not just an information gathering exercise but also the opportunity to begin to form a therapeutic relationship and a basis to establish the trust on which future work can proceed. Therefore, in addition to comprehensively assessing Angela's full range of needs, the CPN also focused on developing a rapport and promoting Angela's confidence. A further important consideration was the assessment of risk as Angela has a young child and therefore their needs are of paramount concern.

From the assessment it emerged that Angela had a number of worries over different situations and felt anxious for much of the time. The main problems were:

* her finances;
* that her partner was unemployed;
* guilt over putting her daughter into nursery when she was at work;
* sleeping difficulties.

While these worries were the same as those Angela confided in the GP, it is important as part of the collaborative relationship to frequently check with the person which needs they most prioritize. This is because people's circumstances can change but also, in the case of a person with GAD, the person frequently has multiple worries and those about which they are most concerned might change. Furthermore, the person may not feel sufficiently confident to volunteer this information and may lose confidence in the therapeutic relationship if the healthcare professional insists on working on a need which they no longer feel to be a priority. It is also important to permit the person to prioritize their needs in order to empower them and place them at the centre of their care.

The CPN explained that they could see Angela for up to six sessions with an evaluation and then the possibility of a further six sessions. Each session would last for up to 50 minutes and consist of a jointly agreed **agenda** at the beginning, and **homework** would be agreed for Angela to complete between sessions. It is helpful when working with a person with GAD to provide a clear definition of the working relationship and to remain consistent as often the person's concentration is affected and therefore keeping to clear **boundaries** is helpful. The deep uncertainty the person can feel can be helped by having the support of a stable therapeutic relationship. Angela agreed to work with the CPN although was uncertain that she could make a change.

INTERVENTION

Following assessment at the next session with Angela, the CPN asked her to rate each of the above areas of worry on a scale of 1–10, with 1 being the lowest. Angela struggled to apply scores to her worries, and so the CPN suggested that she carry out this activity as homework before the next session.

Gaining an indication of the rating of Angela's worries serves several purposes by doing the following:

- allowing the CPN to appreciate how Angela perceives her worries;
- providing useful baseline information against which future ratings of the same concerns can be compared to identify improvement;
- equipping Angela with a rational technique to be able to measure her worry and therefore prioritize her needs, which will help her to focus her efforts and avoid being overwhelmed by her worries.

In order to help Angela to understand her anxiety, the CPN asked her to explain how she felt when she became anxious. Angela stated that everything began to feel as though it was happening very quickly, and the level of her concern spiralled out of control, leading to her experiencing the physical effects of rapid heartbeat, sweating, a knotted feeling in her stomach, and a sense of agitation. Using a whiteboard to draw a simple diagram, the CPN explained that our thoughts affect how we feel, and **negative thoughts** are highly influential in this process, yet can be based on a mistaken interpretation of the events. To illustrate negative thoughts, the CPN identified some different thinking styles. While there are many others, those which the CPN outlined were:

- **All or nothing thinking** – whereby if the person does not succeed completely, then they have failed and there is nothing between these criteria.
- **Negative self-labelling** – focusing on negative personality traits.
- Disqualifying positives – only counting instances which support a negative view.
- **Catastrophization** – believing the worst possible outcome of any given situation.

The CPN discussed with Angela whether she could identify any situations she had experienced where she had applied a negative thinking style. Angela recognized that her concern over making mistakes at work, leading to her losing her job and further worsening her money worries, was an example of catastrophic thinking.

The CPN then suggested that once we have identified our negative thoughts, it is possible to adopt alternative ones which will positively influence how we feel. Angela was not confident that she could change her thoughts, although was keen to identify her negative thinking. Therefore the CPN suggested that Angela keep **thought records** as homework and explained how this technique works. This technique involves the person considering their thoughts in relation to difficult situations, and then identifying their negative thinking, and the effects of these on their feelings. Table 7.1 presents Angela's thought record as she focused on identifying her negative thoughts. The information in thought records varies depending on their intended purpose. For example, Angela did not feel that she could change her thoughts, and so the thought record she used only sought to identify the negative thoughts. Some that are more ambitious aim to develop new thoughts.

In collaborating with Angela, the CPN was aware of the necessity of progressing at a pace at which she felt comfortable and of actively negotiating the interventions in which Angela wished to engage. In promoting her confidence and self-esteem, it was important to provide her with choices and alternatives wherever possible, to allow her to make the choices which reflect her preferences in participating in her treatment.

Angela attended the next session with a number of entries on her thought record and discussed these with the CPN. She found the additional insight which this provided to be useful and continued to keep the thought records over further weeks. However, Angela explained that while she realized that some of the negative thoughts contributing to her anxiety were mistaken, she still found it very difficult to break the spiral of anxiety once it began. Often behaviours are hard to change due to being firmly established and ingrained and therefore change occurs gradually in incremental stages.

As Angela had suggested at the beginning of the session that she was still experiencing problems sleeping, this was also included in the agenda. The CPN provided several sources of information. These included:

- A leaflet on sleep hygiene, covering a range of considerations from creating a suitable environment in which to sleep to recommending actions and patterns of behaviour which would promote rest and sleep.
- Information on relaxation tapes and DVDs.
- An explanation and demonstration of progressive muscle relaxation (Figure 7.1).

At the beginning of the session, Angela also said that she felt that the issue which was causing her most worry at that moment was her finances. The CPN suggested using problem solving. This technique functions by clearly identifying the problem and then generating as wide a range of solutions as possible before considering each option in turn in terms of feasibility and appropriateness to the problem.

In discussion with the CPN it emerged that Angela was **avoiding** dealing with the finances rather than these being the problem due to apprehension over the possible scale of the problem. The CPN identified that Angela had a fairly clear, rational understanding of her financial situation but the belief supporting her anxiety was that her finances were in a bad state. When asked which was the more realistic appraisal, Angela identified that her rational understanding was more likely and she had chosen to avoid dealing with her finances as this was a task which she did not enjoy. The CPN emphasized to Angela that negative thinking can influence how we feel and that in this example she was allowing her negative thoughts about

Table 7.1 Angela's thought record

The situation	First thought	Negative thought	Negative belief	Evidence for and against
An anxiety-provoking situation	Initial thought in the situation	The type of negative thinking	Identify the negative belief	What evidence supports or disproves this view?
Monday morning – Dropping child at nursery	I'm a bad mother	Negative self-labelling	Mothers need to be there for their children	**For** A child needs their parents I miss my child when at work **Against** I need to work I am there for my child at most other times
Thursday evening – Going for a meal with a friend	I should not spend money	All or nothing thinking	I need to be excessively frugal with money	**For** Our finances are stretched I could spend the money on something else **Against** I need some leisure Our bills are all paid
Tuesday morning – Mistake at work	I will lose my job	Catastrophization	I am not good enough to do my job	**For** I have made other mistakes I did not always make mistakes **Against** I have been in my job for a long while without problems before I have the qualifications to do the job Other people have commented positively on my performance

- In a quiet place, make yourself comfortable and close your eyes.
- Tense all of the facial muscles for eight seconds while inhaling.
- Exhale and relax the muscles.
- Repeat the process for the following areas of the body:
  - neck and shoulders
  - chest
  - stomach
  - upper right arm
  - lower right arm
  - right hand
  - upper left arm
  - lower left arm
  - left hand
  - buttocks
  - upper right leg
  - lower right leg
  - right foot
  - upper left leg
  - lower left leg
  - left foot

Figure 7.1 Progressive muscle relaxation

her finances to influence her behaviour making her avoid dealing with the finances which compounded the problem, making her feelings worse.

In addition to continuing to keep the thought records, Angela identified checking her finances as her homework before the next session as a **behavioural experiment**. The CPN suggested that Angela rate her fear before and after the activity. In the next session Angela reported that she had been able to assess and organize her finances. Her level of fear before-hand was reduced due to the discussion with the CPN in the previous session. Also on finding that her finances were not as bad as she had feared but consistent with her rational appraisal of the situation, her overall level of fear throughout the behavioural experiment was less than she had anticipated. By going through her finances Angela felt more empowered and confident in dealing with a problem which she had previously avoided.

Angela continued to work well with the CPN and to identify other issues to address. Most importantly among these were her concerns over her relationship with her daughter. Angela was concerned that her daughter resented her placing her in nursery when she went to work. However, in discussion with the CPN, Angela realized that due to feeling under time pressure, little of her time was spent being with her daughter. She therefore allocated time each week to spend playing with her daughter and was surprised at how much the little girl valued being with her mum. This led Angela to reappraise her negative thoughts and to realize that her feelings that her daughter might resent her really stemmed from her own guilt about placing her daughter in nursery.

Angela attended all 12 sessions with the CPN and engaged in other therapeutic work and made gradual progress. When working with people with GAD, the therapeutic approach adopted needs to be flexible in relation to the person's need and the way in which they experience the problem and to work at their preferred pace.

Angela's partner is still seeking work but they are considering having another child as they would like their daughter to have a sibling close to her age. Angela feels that her anxiety has improved and although she still often feels anxious, the techniques which she has learned have helped her gain in confidence and self-esteem and permit her to challenge the issues in relation to which she feels anxious. Often where people have multiple problems, learning skills to manage some specific problems provides the techniques and confidence to tackle other issues. Angela feels better able to manage her worries and is more optimistic about the future. Before ending the sessions the CPN discussed relapse prevention, and together with Angela identified how she might notice signs of relapse and actions which she might take in these circumstances to access support.

CONCLUSION

People such as Angela experience GAD as severely debilitating, life-limiting and a cause of significant distress to the person and their family and significant others. Working with a person with GAD requires flexibility to focus on the concerns which the person prioritizes and to proceed at their pace while empowering and promoting the person's interests. The use of a CBT-led approach can provide the structure and effective methods to counter negative thoughts and challenge feelings of anxiety. However, establishing effective and trusting therapeutic relationships with clearly defined boundaries and expectations is pivotal in developing the necessary trust and confidence for the person to make sustained and meaningful change. Often people with GAD will experience further problems at challenging times in the future and it is important to ensure that the person has a relapse plan and is readily able to access support.

REFERENCES

McManus, S., Meltzer, H., Brugha, T., Bebbington, P. and Jenkins, R. (2009) *Adult Psychiatric Morbidity in England, 2007: Results of a Household Survey.* London: National Centre for Social Research.

NCCMH (National Collaborating Centre for Mental Health) (2011) *The NICE Guidelines on Management in Primary, Secondary and Community Care: Generalised Anxiety Disorder in Adults.* London: The British Psychological Society and The Royal College of Psychiatrists.

NHS Choices (2011) *Do I Have an Anxiety Disorder?* Available at: http://www.nhs.uk/chq/Pages/2427.aspx (accessed 17 November 2011).

Patient.co.uk (2011) *Generalised Anxiety Disorder.* Available at: http://www.patient.co.uk/health/Anxiety-Generalised-Anxiety-Disorder.htm (accessed 17 November 2011).

CASE STUDY 8
Depression
Nick Wrycraft

Laura is a 46-year-old married mother of three children, experiencing depression. She has begun to feel low in mood over the past three months and has visited her GP who prescribed anti-depressant medication and referred her to a mental health nurse (RMN) who liaises with the surgery. The RMN used some of the principles from a cognitive behavioural therapy (CBT) approach to inform her work, including agenda setting, homework and the therapeutic techniques of **activity scheduling,** sleep hygiene and progressive muscle relaxation.

The mental health nurse used a structured assessment in order to gain a detailed understanding of Laura's background, current circumstances and mental state. The areas the assessment considered included:

- her presentation in the interview;
- activities and social life;
- family;
- mood;
- nutrition;
- sleep;
- risk.

BACKGROUND

Laura was born in an African country and moved to the UK with her parents and sister, who is two years older than her, when she was 5 years old. Her mother had been a primary school teacher and Laura's father was a policeman. To her parents' disappointment, however, they had difficulty finding work in these professions, and so her mother stayed at home looking after the family and her father eventually found employment at a factory making electronic equipment.

Laura describes her early life and childhood as difficult because the family had very little money and struggled financially. Laura and her sister did not get the same expensive presents at birthdays and Christmas as many of their friends, and they often wore second-hand or cheap clothes which made Laura feel embarrassed and ashamed. Laura describes her parents as being deeply religious and principled and very keen for Laura and her sister to succeed and make a good life to the extent that her mother carried out many hours of extra schoolwork with her daughters.

Laura says that her sister was very successful academically and socially popular. Laura tried very hard but struggled at school, and was quiet and made few friends and feels that she has always lacked self-esteem and confidence. While her sister went to a good university, Laura became convinced that she would not achieve her parents' aspirations and be a disappointment and was very upset when she only narrowly achieved the required grades for university. She identifies this experience as triggering her first episode of depression, whereby she had a sustained low mood for several months. Laura was prescribed anti-depressants by her GP and had a brief number of sessions with a therapist in cognitive behavioural therapy (CBT). Laura says that she did not find these useful as she did not find the therapist to be very understanding and empathic.

While at university Laura met her future husband, gained a good degree and then moved to a city where she had a successful working career until the birth of her first child after which she experienced post-natal depression (PND), for which she was again prescribed anti-depressants and was supported by her health visitor. Feeling unable to return to her job, Laura and her husband moved to a small town and had two more children but Laura did not experience any further instances of PND.

As her children grew up, Laura worked in several part-time jobs through an employment agency to fit in with caring for her family. She feels that her current experience of depression occurred following the end of a temporary job which she particularly enjoyed and was disappointed to have ended, and since then the agency has had difficulty finding her further work. At the same time, her eldest son has struggled at school and been refusing to attend. Laura is very concerned that she is now experiencing depression in response to smaller and smaller events, and worried that her future life will consist of repeated episodes of depression.

CURRENT EXPERIENCE OF DEPRESSION

Presentation

Laura lacked animation when speaking and did not initiate conversation, only responding to questions which the nurse asked and appeared very tired, **lethargic** and unmotivated. Laura avoided eye contact and was dressed in baggy, dark-coloured clothing and looked unkempt.

Activities and social life

Laura has a few close friends whom she has known for a long while and finds very supportive. She is reluctant to mix with people she does not know well as she believes that they will realize she is depressed and dislike her. Laura also often feels inadequate and compares herself negatively to other people. Even though she is aware that she does this, Laura feels unable to challenge these thoughts and they worsen her mood. As a result, she has also stopped doing many of her usual activities, including evening classes, going to the gym and is socializing less with her friends. Laura also describes having lost interest in reading and watching television. Instead she says that she feels as though she has no interests, and does not know what to do with her time.

Family

Her husband works long hours and often has to go on trips away from home, which means that Laura has to take a lot of responsibility for the family, and worries about making wrong decisions. When her husband is at home, he is often tired, or has to deal with work-related phone calls or emails. Laura does not like to bother him with issues concerning the children as she feels that these seem trivial in relation to his work. Due to her husband's frequent absences and her low mood Laura says that their sex life has reduced significantly. She feels isolated and unsupported yet unable to communicate these feelings to her husband. Although Laura describes the family as having a close relationship, her children are aged 17, 14 and 12 and have become increasingly independent and she no longer feels needed.

Mood

Laura says that she has felt very low in mood almost all of the time for the past three months, and often experiences negative thoughts. When asked to rate her current mood from 1 to 10, with 1 being the lowest, she identifies her mood today as 3. Laura says that she does not feel motivated to do things and lacks confidence, experiencing negative and self-critical thoughts. For example, she recently put some laundry in the washing machine but inadvertently did not check the temperature and the clothes were ruined, for which Laura blamed herself. Since then Laura asks her children to do the washing, disguising the real reason for asking by suggesting this is a method of their earning extra money. Laura does not buy clothes for herself due to her mood and self-esteem.

Nutrition

Often the family eat separately, and due to her low mood, Laura misses meals. She feels that she has lost a lot of weight over recent months reducing as much as two clothes sizes.

Sleep

Laura explained that she cannot sleep at night, often remaining awake for long periods of time, feeling anxious and restless. As a result of being tired in the morning, she stays in bed during the day with the curtains closed because she 'cannot face the world'.

Risk

Laura says that she has no plans to end her life although often feels as though she no longer wants to live. She feels that she could never express this in front of her children.

1 **What is depression?**

A Depression is the most common mental health problem (NCCMH 2011). It is characterized by the loss of enjoyment of life and is evident when the person functions differently to how they are normally for at least two weeks, and for most of every day in a range of areas, including behaviour, cognitions, emotions, physical factors (APA 1994; NICE 2009; NCCMH 2011).

Among the features of depression are:
Behaviour:

- avoidance of others;
- withdrawal from social activities and friendships;
- not engaging in self-care, and self-neglect.

Cognitions:

- negative thoughts;
- self-critical thoughts and negative self-appraisal;
- reduced and slowed-down ability to think, inability to concentrate or make decisions;
- recurrent thoughts of death, self-harm or suicidal ideation most of the time.

Emotions:

- low mood and absence of feeling or feeling detached; alternatively the person may be very tearful;
- feelings of worthlessness, hopelessness, self-loathing, low self-esteem or guilt.

Physical factors:

- significantly reduced interest and motivation in all, or almost all activities for the majority of the time nearly every day;
- decreased activity;
- feelings of fatigue and a lack of energy and interest;
- significant unplanned weight loss (5 per cent of total body weight within a month, or the equivalent) or weight gain;
- insomnia or hypersomnia;
- loss of interest in sex.

There is a high rate of co-morbidity with depression also commonly occurring alongside other health problems. For example:

- alcohol or substance misuse;
- another mental health problem, for example, personality disorder, schizophrenia, obsessive compulsive disorder (OCD), or post-traumatic stress disorder (PTSD);
- pain due to a physical health problem;
- a life-limiting physical health problem.

2 **Which of the above are evident in Laura's case?**

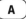 **A**
- Laura's behaviour avoided engagement by only responding to questions and not making eye contact.
- Laura has experienced a low mood for a sustained period of time with a reduction in interest in the activities which she used to pursue.
- Negative thoughts.
- General lack of energy and interest.
- Missing meals and weight loss.
- Disrupted sleeping pattern (insomnia).
- Loss of interest in sex.
- Feelings of low worth and low self-esteem when comparing herself to others.
- Laura has not contemplated suicide but has wished that she were not alive any more.

Everyone experiences depression differently and the presence of even a few features can significantly impair the person's quality of life (NICE 2009). In assessing the extent of severity of a person's depression, it is important to consider carefully the following:

- How long has the person been experiencing these features?
- To what extent is their life impaired by their problem?
- How disabling is the problem?
- What effect is their problem having on their family/social network?
- What support might the person's family/social network provide?

3 **What causes depression?**

A Depression is present in all cultures and populations (NCCMH 2011). There are biological, psychological and sociological explanations for the cause of depression.

- From a biological perspective, the fact that anti-depressant medication is effective is often assumed as evidence that there is a physiological cause. Often members of the same family also experience depression which might indicate a genetic component.
- However, this has also been interpreted as support of the psychological explanation for depression, on the rationale that we learn behaviours from people who are influential in our lives, even if these are negative coping mechanisms.
- The sociological explanation of depression suggests that if we experience detrimental living circumstances, this is likely although not inevitable to increase our predisposition to experiencing depression.

Nationally and internationally, there is a higher incidence of depression in women than men and among people from minority ethnic backgrounds (NCCMH 2011). The reasons for the greater prevalence among women is not known, although in the UK the factors which might contribute include:

- Women seek contact with the health services more than men and are more likely to be in contact with health professionals who might identify depression. Most obviously women are in contact through the maternity services.

- As is the case with Laura, many women are often carers, and take responsible roles within the family which can expose them to emotional stressors causing depression.
- It has been suggested that some health services are more likely to regard women as depressed than men, reflecting a gender bias in diagnosing depression.
- Increasingly, in recent decades, there is the expectation that women will have successful working careers and children which imposes pressures and high expectations on women.
- It is still the case that women earn less than men and inequalities within society can mean that women do not receive the same opportunities as men to achieve their aspirations.

4   **What is the recommended treatment for depression?**

A   There are a number of evidence-based interventions recommended for people with depression. These include:

- Psychological interventions:
  - Cognitive behavioural therapy (CBT);
  - Activity scheduling;
  - **Interpersonal therapy (IPT);**
  - Mindfulness-based cognitive therapy (NCCMH 2011);
  - Computerized CBT;
- Self-help literature (NICE 2009).

In the case of people with moderate to severe depression, medication might also be considered. There are a number of anti-depressant medications available including:

- selective serotonin reuptake inhibitors (SSRIs);
- **tricyclics (TCAs)**;
- **monoamine oxidase inhibitors (MAOIs).**

Other interventions include:

- counselling;
- peer and family support;
- self-help groups.

Electroconvulsive therapy (ECT) is still used. However, in recent years this has declined with the development of increasingly effective forms of treatment. ECT is only recommended where other treatments have not succeeded, and the person's quality of life remains deeply affected by their depression.

The option or combination of therapeutic options used will vary depending on the person's preferences and circumstances. However, the choice of treatment needs to be discussed and agreed collaboratively between the healthcare practitioner and the person, and to reflect careful consideration of the nature of the person's problem and their preferences.

5 **Which interventions might benefit Laura?**

A Laura is already taking anti-depressant medication prescribed by her GP. At the end of the assessment she agreed to attend one-to-one sessions with the RMN at the GP's surgery each week. The mental health nurse asked Laura to carry out some homework over the week, and to attend the next session with a list of issues which she prioritized, and wanted to improve in her life.

The RMN began the sessions which followed with Laura by agreeing an agenda of issues to discuss. Agenda setting permits equal participation between the person and the healthcare professional. This is consistent with a CBT approach whereby the person is expected to participate actively in their treatment which fosters empowerment and, in Laura's case, will be helpful to promote her self-esteem.

When Laura attended the next session, the list of issues which she had prioritized included:

- for her mood to improve;
- to be able to have a better sleep pattern;
- to improve her relationship with her husband.

Laura and the RMN discussed how these priorities might be interpreted and made into goals, beginning with improving her mood. Laura's lack of activity was discussed and she felt that the less she did, the worse she felt and the more her confidence eroded. Laura felt that being more active in the daytime would help her mood through gaining some sense of achievement.

At the RMN's suggestion, Laura agreed to carry out activity scheduling which is often effective in helping people who lack motivation, and consists of the person prioritizing tasks (BBC n.d.). This technique is carried out in different ways and frequently adapted; however, one way in which activities can be grouped are as:

- pleasurable;
- involving a sense of achievement;
- involving physical activity;
- involving social activity.

The range of activities reflects the varied tasks we undertake in everyday life, and in considering how to combine these, it is advisable to balance those which represent a challenge with those we find pleasurable.

Laura and the RMN identified and agreed activities which fitted these areas, and then wrote them on the diary sheet. Laura chose to phone a friend she knew well and felt comfortable seeing, but whom she had not been in contact with for some months, to arrange to meet as a social activity later in the week. Putting away the laundry and vacuuming the house were activities which she identified as providing a sense of achievement. Laura also agreed to write down how she felt after completing the activities. She was wary of identifying too many as she did not feel confident. However, the nurse reassured Laura that it was best to progress at a gradual pace at which she felt comfortable. For some people with significant motivation issues, using a smaller activity sheet might help the person not to feel daunted by the list.

At the next session with the RMN, Laura reported some success. The added structure which the activity schedule gave her was useful (see Table 8.1), while she felt that identifying

Table 8.1 Example of an activity schedule

	Pleasurable activity	Activity with a sense of achievement	Physical activity	Social activity
Monday				
Tuesday				
Wednesday				
Thursday				
Friday				
Saturday				
Sunday				

Source: Adapted from BBC, *Headroom* (n.d.).

specific tasks helped her to focus her motivation. Laura's sleep was then discussed. Although Laura is experiencing depression, people also often co-morbidly experience anxiety. For Laura, this often occurred at night as a result of **ruminating** or dwelling upon her negative thoughts. The nurse introduced sleep hygiene, explaining that this involves the environment and practice of sleeping, and includes the following procedures. To change the environment, Laura was advised to do the following:

- remove the television or computer from the bedroom;
- ensure that the room is suitably ventilated;
- within economic constraints, decorate the room in colours and furnishings which promote relaxation;
- keep the bedroom dark by, for example, using blinds or curtains which do not permit light to enter;
- ensure that the pillows, mattress and bedcovers are comfortable.

The practice of sleeping is as follows:

- Go to bed at approximately the same time each night.
- Have a regular pattern of behaviour or routine before going to bed which focuses on gradually increasing relaxation and activities which do not require significant mental activity.
- Avoid eating large meals late in the evening, though if hungry, eat a light non-spicy or non-sugary snack.
- Avoid alcohol or drinks which contain stimulants such as coffee, tea or energy drinks for at least four hours before going to bed.
- If unable to sleep, get up and watch television, read or listen to the radio and return to bed when tired.

While many of these measures might seem obvious, often experiencing an inability to sleep and anxiety, can cause people to overlook simple problem-solving measures. Laura was surprised that she had not considered that remaining in bed worrying about not sleeping did not resolve the issue. Instead she agreed with the nurse that if she had trouble sleeping, she would listen to the radio, as she had stopped watching television or reading. Laura's home-work was to write down when she went to bed and woke up again, any interruptions with her sleep and to rate how rested she felt on waking.

When reporting back in the next session, Laura found that there had been some improve-ment with her sleeping over the week, but that she still tended to wake up in the night feeling anxious. Listening to the radio until she felt tired and then returning to bed was an effective technique but Laura still woke up tired. The RMN suggested that Laura write down the situ-ation she felt anxious about to try and quantify her worry, and to try to generate positive solutions and resolve to deal with the problem in the morning.

As a further measure to encourage sleep, the RMN explained the technique of progressive muscle relaxation, whereby the person tenses groups of muscles in their body as they breathe in and then relaxes them as they breathe out (see Figure 7.1 on p. 59). In discussion with Laura it was agreed that avoiding going to bed during the day might help her sleep at night, and that carrying out physical activity such as exercise can help with sleep. To achieve this goal, Laura increased the tasks she carried out in the activity schedule. Laura's sleep improved gradually over several weeks which is not uncommon as sleep is determined by routine changing patterns which can often take time to establish.

Although progress was not without hindrances, by engaging in simple tasks and using activity scheduling, Laura felt her confidence and sense of achievement grow. The RMN noticed that over the weeks Laura's mood had improved and she engaged in the one-to-one sessions to a greater extent. Establishing a working collaborative relationship and sense of trust is pivotal in determining the outcome of psychological interventions.

In further sessions with the RMN Laura agreed to focus upon improving her relationship with her husband. Laura identified several goals which she would like to achieve:

- to spend more time with her husband;
- to be able to share some of her feelings about being isolated and unsupported;
- to discuss the future with her husband now that the children were more independent.

Laura and her husband did not have a wide range of people to ask who might be able to provide child care. Also when the children were younger, Laura found it stressful to leave them, and so preferred simply not to go out very often which has endured for several years, leading to her rarely being alone to speak with her husband. The nurse suggested that as the children are older now, they might be able to manage at home alone for an evening. Laura agreed that she might be able to arrange an evening out with her husband.

In the next session Laura reported that she had arranged an evening out with her husband but was concerned about sharing her feelings with her husband and her wish to discuss the future fearing that: 'it might come out all wrong'. The RMN suggested using **behavioural rehearsal**, whereby she assumed the role of Laura's husband and Laura put her feelings and thoughts into words. This allowed Laura to reflect on her thoughts and consider how she might articulate these feelings to her husband. Laura was able to express how she felt to her husband and realized that her anxiety around these feelings was disproved as he responded very positively and was keen to make changes to improve their family life.

CONCLUSION

Laura was funded by her GP for 12 sessions with the RMN during which time her mood lifted, she became more active, her sleep pattern improved and she also felt that she had begun to re-establish a relationship with her husband. Unfortunately, like many people, Laura has experienced depression on more than one occasion in her life, and the more episodes the person has, the more likely are further instances to recur. Often these are in response to stressors or detrimental life events. However, relapse is not always inevitable and Laura's fear that she would continue to experience depression in response to less and less significant stressful factors is not necessarily the case. When working with people with depression, it is important to carefully consider how to optimize strengths and positive coping resources in order to promote their resilience and minimize the possibility of relapse.

When coming towards the end of her sessions with the RMN, and discussing how she might avoid relapse, Laura decided to pay privately for CBT sessions with a therapist. She regarded this as essential to avoid the possibility of relapse by addressing the deep-rooted issues and ingrained beliefs which began in her childhood relating to her low self-esteem and confidence and which now contribute to her negative thoughts and self-appraisal, and her act of making detrimental self-comparisons with other people. While this work is challenging and ongoing, Laura feels that she has gained skills in problem-solving, and the nurse's style of working introduced and acquainted Laura to some important aspects of the CBT model which she will find useful in the future.

REFERENCES

American Psychiatric Association (2000) *Diagnostic and Statistical Manual of Mental Disorders*, 4th edn, text revision. Washington, DC: APA.

BBC (n. d.) Activity scheduling: the fabulous four, in *Headroom Well-being Guide*. Available at: http://downloads.bbc.co.uk/headroom/cbt/activity_scheduling.pdf (accessed 25 October 2011).

NCCMH (National Collaborating Centre for Mental Health) (2011) *Common Mental Health Disorders: Identification and Pathways to Care*. National Clinical Guideline Number 123. London: NICE.

NICE (National Institute for Health and Clinical Excellence) (2009) *Depression: The Treatment and Management of Depression in Adults*. London: NICE.

CASE STUDY 9
Obsessive compulsive disorder (OCD)
Vanessa Skinner and Nick Wrycraft

Robert is 28 years old and lives at home with his mother and stepfather. His parents divorced when he was 7, which he found very difficult as he felt responsible for protecting his mum emotionally. However, he gets on well with his stepfather, and continues to have a close and supportive relationship with his mum. Robert has no social network and has never had a girlfriend. He describes himself as being very shy. He works as a landscape gardener, which he particularly enjoys due to the physical freedom of being outside, and because he has an interest in nature. Robert thinks he has high standards, and describes himself as a perfectionist, often seeking reassurance that he has got things 'just right'.

Four years ago he experienced a period of depression which improved following treatment with anti-depressant medication. However, his current difficulty began four months ago when he started to experience distressing intrusive thoughts that he had unknowingly hit someone while driving.

These intrusive thoughts were originally triggered when a gust of wind caught his van, making a loud thumping sound just as he was passing a person standing on the hard shoulder. Robert was alone at the time, and as the journey continued, he became obsessed with the thought that he had hit the person. He described experiencing feelings of anxiety and guilt and felt compelled to retrace his route to check.

Since then, whenever Robert is driving, any loud sound, such as going over a pothole or drain, triggers the same intrusive thoughts, feelings of guilt and the compulsion to check that he has not accidentally hit someone. Robert is also aware that if he notices a drift in his concentration when driving, or has difficulty recalling the exact route he has taken, he experiences these same feelings of doubt and uncertainty and feels the compulsion to check that he has not hit someone without realizing it.

Travelling to and from work took him a long time due to his constant compulsion to retrace his journey and check that he had not hit someone, eventually requiring him to leave home very early in the morning and still often arrive very late for work. This eventually became so stressful that Robert stopped driving on his own, and his mum started to accompany him to and from work, which he found embarrassing in front of his colleagues. However, he didn't tell anyone about the problem, believing that he might lose his job if people knew.

Robert was referred for CBT by a mental health nurse practitioner attached to his GP's surgery. He had difficulty making sense of his problem and at assessment initially appeared anxious and self-conscious. However, by the end of the session he expressed relief at being able to talk about the problem and to find that it was 'normal' behaviour for a person experiencing obsessive compulsive disorder (OCD).

What are the features of OCD?

A Obsessive compulsive disorder (OCD) involves the presence of **obsessions** or **compulsions**, and commonly both, which the person recognizes as imposing excessive demands upon them, and upsetting their everyday life. OCD places a significant burden upon the person in terms of emotional distress and loss of quality of life. The APA (2000) suggest that a person may be experiencing OCD if the focus of their obsessions and compulsions requires in excess of one hour a day, although for many people these will occupy a significantly greater amount of their time.

OBSESSIONS

Obsessions are experienced as intrusive thoughts, images or urges which are persistent and unwanted, and which cause significant anxiety or distress. Although the person may have insight and know these thoughts are produced by their mind, and not caused by the environment around them, and also be aware that they place an unreasonable demand or burden upon them, they are unable to prevent their occurrence (APA 2000; NCCMH 2011). However, the person will often engage in attempts to distract themselves from the obsessive thoughts, or use other methods such as **safety behaviours** to reduce their effects.

Among the frequent themes for obsessions are:

- contamination by, for example, dirt or germs;
- excessive preoccupation with illness or physical symptoms;
- fear of harm, such as forgetting to turn off electricity or gas;
- concern with order or symmetry;
- hoarding useless or worthless items;
- religious, sacrilegious or blasphemous thoughts;
- sexual thoughts relating to deviancy;
- thoughts of violence or aggression.

COMPULSIONS

Compulsions are repetitive behaviours or mental acts which the person feels compelled to perform in connection with their obsessive thoughts in order to reduce distress, or to prevent a feared outcome (APA 2000; NCCMH 2011). However, in spite of the function of compulsive acts being to reduce distress, they are not pleasurable experiences, as there is no reward, only the prevention of the feared outcome, which is often followed by further occurrences of obsessive thoughts. Many people with OCD will also feel shame or guilt as they do not wish to perform the compulsions, and experience a sense of a loss of self-determination or volition.

Compulsions can be **overt** and readily observed by others, for example, physical behaviours, or **covert** in the form of mental acts which are not visible.

Frequent themes for compulsions include:

- excessive and elaborate cleaning rituals;
- excessive attention to personal hygiene, for example, bathing and personal hygiene;

- repeated checking, for example, domestic appliances, plug sockets and doors;
- placing objects in a very specific order, or symmetrical pattern;
- collecting and hoarding items with little value or worth;
- special words or phrases repeated in a specific order;
- counting.

2 **Consider your own experience of persistent thoughts, or those of people you know that might be regarded as obsessive. How might this feel?**

A Although the obsessive thoughts and compulsive acts involved in OCD often appear to be strange, or to defy logical explanation, the most commonly occurring compulsions are checking and cleaning (NCCMH 2011). It is believed that this is because they relate to everyday activities which we all carry out, and that OCD is an exaggeration of concerns which are normal, and experienced by a large proportion of the population (NCCMH 2011). However, for some people, this becomes a pervasive concern and the emotional distress and time consumed ruminating over obsessive thoughts and the performance of compulsive actions mean that OCD is experienced as much more acute and life-dominating in contrast with our own passing experiences.

3 **How would you explain Robert's experience of OCD?**

A In seeking to understand Robert's experience of OCD, research by Salkovskis and Harrison (1984, cited in Salkovskis 1999) indicates that intrusive thoughts are a normal phenomenon among the general population. However, in OCD, the person interprets these signals as meaning that they have a personal responsibility for harm and its prevention. Checking behaviours are a key feature of the disorder, and used by the person on the rationale of their either preventing or neutralizing harm or in response to a perceived responsibility (Salkovskis, cited in Tarrier et al. 1999). In Robert's case, when driving, he interprets his intrusive thoughts to mean that he might be responsible for harm, which profoundly increases his sense of responsibility and guilt.

Another understanding of Robert's experience of OCD is offered by Freeston et al. (1996), where responsibility is also regarded as a factor, but also the over-estimation of threat, perfectionism and intolerance of uncertainty. Robert recognizes himself as a perfectionist; when driving, he experienced anxiety over the uncertainty and needed to check in order to make sure, yet still was unable to resolve his doubts.

Robert also over-estimated negative thoughts, by believing that he was likely to cause an accident unless he constantly acted to prevent this outcome, hence his concern at any loss of total concentration. This inflated sense of responsibility resulted in him taking every possible action to prevent his feared consequence, and he could not tolerate any loss of concentration, as this would mean uncertainty, and would trigger the assumption, 'I must have hit someone.'

The urgency of the obsessive thought can also influence a person's interpretation of its importance in a concept known as 'thought–action–fusion' (Rachman 1993, cited in Wells 1997: 239). This is based on the premise that the emotions accompanying a thought can influence the person's interpretation of its meaning. In Robert's case, the strength of the feeling accompanying the thought that he has hit a person when driving leads him to conclude that this has been the case. As a result of this, Robert experiences guilt, and a feeling that he has done something wrong, and subsequent anxiety through basing his appraisal of the situation on a negative emotional response (Wills and Sanders 1997).

4   **How might we begin working with Robert?**

A   All therapeutic work begins with assessing the problem and establishing the basis for a collaborative relationship between the healthcare worker and person. A CBT assessment was carried out with Robert, and this involved gathering specific information regarding the problem, including identifying triggers, thoughts, physical responses, emotions and behaviours. The problem was then conceptualized using a **formulation**, explaining how the various aspects of the problem fitted together and maintained the difficulty (Westbrook et al. 2007).

When working with Robert and people who experience OCD, because the person seeks to resist the obsessive thoughts and reduce their fears, it is important to recognize and explore the effect of the preventative or neutralizing behaviours which the person has used to keep them 'safe' in the short term. Robert identified that the technique he used when driving was to check the mirrors around six or seven times a minute.

However, as is often the case with safety behaviours, while helping to make the person feel safer in the short term, there is a paradoxical effect in the long term of maintaining the problem by increasing preoccupation with the concern, which in turn prompts further intrusive thoughts. Also, by checking so frequently in the mirror, Robert increased the likelihood of his experiencing the feared event of having an accident, as he was not concentrating on the road ahead (Salkovskis and McGuire, cited in Menzies and de Silva 2003: 64).

Robert believed that by driving very carefully and continually checking, he could prevent his feared consequence from happening, which negatively reinforced these behaviours and maintained the problem. If he experienced doubt, he would try to drive even more carefully and check more, making matters worse (Hawton et al. 1989).

Robert's mum was keen to support him and became involved in his safety behaviours by agreeing to accompany him wherever he drove. While Robert found that her presence and verbal reassurance reduced his anxiety in the short term, in the longer term, his reliance on her support reduced his personal confidence when driving, and increased the difficulty of his being able to drive alone in the future. It was therefore helpful, with Robert's consent, to provide his mum with some CBT literature designed for relatives of people with OCD explaining how they can really be of help, by encouraging the person to value their own judgement rather than continue to offer them reassurance (Hyman and Pedrick 1999; NICE 2005).

5   **What treatment might be suitable for Robert?**

A   NICE guidelines (2005) recommend the CBT technique of **exposure and response prevention (ERP)** as the treatment of choice for people with OCD. This involves the person facing their feared situation without employing their safety behaviours. However, ERP often appears daunting for people when OCD symptoms are at their worst. Instead optimum treatment for some may include medication initially, followed by ERP (NICE 2005). Robert had been prescribed and was taking the anti-depressant medication **citalopram**.

Each person's problem is experienced differently, and when working in psychological therapy it is necessary to establish a therapeutic rapport and to clarify the expectations of each party and to jointly agree with the person their priorities for therapeutic work. Robert's perfectionism contributed to the problem he experienced with driving, and was potentially an issue in his work with the CBT therapist, as he was inclined to set goals which were too high, or to expect unattainable standards of both himself and the therapist. At the end of the assessment, the therapist tactfully raised this point: 'So, all this checking and reassurance seeking, this is the answer, do you think?'

Framing this thought within a question was a useful technique as it highlighted what might be a sensitive issue but in a less assertive manner than making a statement. This allowed the therapist to work collaboratively with Robert, consistent with the principles of CBT, by encouraging him to question his *own* thoughts and assumptions. Robert responded positively to the question, recognizing that this was a trait which he demonstrated and might need to address.

It was agreed between the therapist and Robert that the aim of his treatment was to establish a 'detached acceptance of intrusive thoughts' (Wells 1997). This was in order to remove the fusion of thoughts and actions which led him to attribute value to thoughts based on the emotional strength by which they were experienced and to assume he had run someone over because he had this thought (Rachman 1993, cited in Wells 1997). The other goals identified were for Robert to be able to drive to work and back on his own, without having to return and check for accidents or seek reassurance from his mum.

Research indicates that OCD responds best to exposure and response prevention (Abramowitz 1996). This involves exposure to the person's feared situation, which invokes anxiety, therefore the specific activity needs to be carefully negotiated and agreed with the person so that they are empowered. It is also important that the person does not respond to their compulsions by engaging in safety behaviours during exposure, as this will dilute the experience and, as with Robert's previous safety behaviours, represents only a short-term solution without remedying the problem (Wells 1997).

Robert agreed to drive on his own around the village for five minutes each day to start with. He chose the village as he knew the area very well, there was less traffic and he felt more in control within this environment. During this time if he felt an urge to check, he agreed to delay his response for at least the time it took him to get back home. He was to record the strength of his urge to check every two minutes until it began to subside. To his surprise, Robert found that, with difficulty, he was able to resist the urge.

After the first week, it was agreed in session that Robert would increase the length of his journeys by five minutes a day. His mood improved and his confidence grew as he did so. By the fourth session he was contemplating driving to work on his own and by the sixth session was driving to work and back independently without returning to check the road.

However, he had started to substitute a new neutralizing behaviour of checking his vehicle for dents and scratches to make sure he hadn't inadvertently hit anyone at the end of each journey. This behaviour increased his compulsive urges and because of this, he believed he had made little real progress. Once he applied the same principles to this new behaviour, the compulsions again subsided.

Robert eventually reached his original target of driving to work and back on his own without returning to check the route. He does not request, and is not given verbal reassurance at any point, and is able to manage his uncertainty without resorting to checking the internet or news for reported accidents. This has led to lifestyle changes, and has given him back his independence. He has joined a dating agency and been offered promotion at work. This has increased his confidence as well as giving him something more productive to spend his time on than the checking.

It was agreed that the remainder of the sessions would focus on the thought–action–fusion aspect of the formulation, while Robert continues with the exposure and response prevention work.

Robert expressed concerns about finishing treatment, and he and the therapist agreed to discuss these over the final few sessions, which were tapered to one a fortnight and eventually one a month. The final sessions included work on relapse prevention. Throughout treatment, Robert has been encouraged to ascribe his progress to personal effort. He has kept a journal to reflect upon his successes, and to record how he dealt with setbacks along the way (Beck 1995). Following treatment, a six-week follow-up session for support and feedback was arranged and things were still going well for him at this point.

REFERENCES

Abramowitz, J.S. (1996) Variants of exposure and response prevention in the treatment of obsessive compulsive disorder: a meta-analysis, *Behaviour Therapy*, 27(4): 583–600.

American Psychiatric Association (2000) *Diagnostic and Statistical Manual of Psychiatric Disorders*, text revision. Washington, DC: APA.

Beck, J. (1995) *Cognitive Therapy: Basics and Beyond*. New York: Guilford Press.

Freeston, M.H., Dugas, M.J. and Ladouceur, R. (1996) Thoughts, images, worry and anxiety, *Cognitive Therapy and Research*, 20: 265–73.

Hawton, K., Salkovskis, P.M., Kirk, J. and Clark, D.M. (1989) *Cognitive Behaviour Therapy for Psychiatric Problems*. Oxford: Oxford University Press.

Hyman, B.M. and Pedrick, C. (1999) *The OCD Workbook, Your Guide to Breaking Free from Obsessive-Compulsive Disorder*. Palo Alto, CA: New Harbinger Publications, Inc.

Menzies, R.G. and de Silva, P. (2003) *Obsessive-Compulsive Disorder: Theory, Research and Treatment*. Chichester: John Wiley & Sons, Ltd.

NCCMH (National Collaborating Centre for Mental Health) (2011) *Common Mental Health Disorders: Identification and Pathways to Care*. National Clinical Guideline Number 123. London: DoH.

NICE (National Institute for Health and Clinical Excellence) (2005) Clinical Guidance 31, *Obsessive Compulsive Disorder (OCD) and Body Dysmorphic Disorder (BDD)*. London: NICE.

Salkovskis, P. (1999) Understanding and treating obsessive-compulsive disorder, *Behaviour Research and Therapy*, 37: 29–52.

Tarrier, N., Wells, A. and Haddock, G. (1999) *Treating Complex Cases: The CBT Approach*. Chichester: John Wiley & Sons, Ltd.

Wells, A. (1997) *Cognitive Therapy of Anxiety Disorders: A Practice Manual and Conceptual Guide*. Chichester: John Wiley & Sons Ltd.

Westbrook, D., Kennerley, H. and Kirk, J. (2007) *An Introduction to Cognitive Behaviour Therapy, Skills and Applications*. London: Sage.

Wills, F. and Sanders, D. (1997) *Cognitive Therapy: Transforming the Image*. London: Sage.

Phobia
Vanessa Skinner and Nick Wrycraft

Lucy is a 28-year-old banking advisor who has been living with her partner for four years. She has been referred by her GP for cognitive behavioural therapy (CBT) due to experiencing fear of vomiting, or **emetophobia**, both regarding herself and other people.

Lucy has managed the problem until now by being careful of her own and her partner's dietary intake, avoiding certain foods and rigidly following the 'use by' dates on food packaging. Lucy also avoids travelling by plane or public transport, is hypervigilant of others and avoids going past pubs and clubs, walking through town at night, crowds, public transport, and anyone who shows signs of being ill.

Lucy has decided to seek help now as she and her partner want to start a family. However, the fear that she might experience morning sickness, together with the thought of having to care for a baby and concerns that it might vomit represent obstacles to achieving that wish. Lucy's GP has referred her to a CBT therapist whom she can see at the GP's surgery.

At the assessment Lucy was highly motivated to overcome her fear. She traced the origin of the problem back to an incident in childhood, when a boy in her class at school suddenly and unexpectedly vomited. The boy was quite close to her and she retains a close recollection of the event. However, she was terrified about what the treatment might involve, and made it clear that she needed to feel 'in control' of things.

1 **What are phobias?**

A Phobias are an anxiety-related condition, and may be present where the person has a significant and persistent fear of a particular object or situation which is disproportionate to the actual level of risk which is present.

The fear and anxiety experienced in phobia are triggered when the person is in the presence of or encounters the particular object or situation, and leads to their trying to avoid it, or experiencing extreme emotional distress if they remain in its presence. Therefore phobias can cause significant inconvenience, leading to people organizing their lives around avoiding the feared object or situation (NCCMH 2011; NHS Choices 2011). In most cases, the person has insight and recognizes that the fear is excessive, yet feels unable to change their response (NCCMH 2011).

2 **Are phobias common?**

A Phobias are very common, with around ten million people in the UK being affected (NHS Choices 2011). While there are many different phobias, they can be regarded as occurring in two groups: **simple phobias** and **complex phobias**:

Simple phobias are where the fear is towards something specific and these are many and varied, for example:

- animals such as dogs, rats, snakes, spiders or insects;
- health-related, for example, being exposed to infection or bodily fluids though fear of contracting an illness;
- risk and well-being, for example, choking, vomiting, fear of needles;
- sensations, such as the feeling of cotton wool, buttons or baked beans;
- situational, for example, heights, flying, being in a lift or on an elevator;
- the natural environment, for example, lightning, storms, thunder or water.

Complex phobias refer to a circumstance or situation, and examples are:

- agoraphobia, or fear of public or open spaces;
- social phobia, or anxiety concerning public situations.

People with agoraphobia often have concerns about leaving their home and being in public situations or open spaces such as shopping centres or public transport. Often there is an associated need to be able to exit a place quickly. In contrast, people with social phobia have anxiety concerning situations such as parties and weddings, and which may also be apparent in a reluctance to speak in front of groups of other people. Often this is due to a fear of public embarrassment. Simple phobias can still be experienced as acutely anxiety-provoking and distressing. Complex phobias often occur later in life and, due to their broader and more pervasive nature, are often deep-rooted. Emetophobia has been identified as more difficult to treat than other specific phobias (Veale 2009).

3 **How do phobias develop?**

A The origin of phobias is not known, as while members of the same families often develop them, this may be a learned rather than genetic response. Also some fears may be innate and natural, for example, relating to spiders, snakes, rats or animals which might do us harm.

Phobias also often develop through experience in early childhood. In Lucy's case, we understand that her belief was triggered when witnessing the boy suddenly and unexpectedly vomit. As a result of this experience, Lucy thinks that in circumstances where this is even remotely possible, it is inevitable that the person will vomit and this fear makes her anxious.

Lucy's response, as is often the case with people who have a phobia, is to adopt safety behaviours or strategies to avoid the feared situation. Yet these actions only worsen the problem as the original fear remains unaddressed.

Frequently simple phobias which develop in childhood disappear over time. However, as in Lucy's case, where the phobia persists into adulthood, the person can experience significant anxiety and distress and the phobia can have severe life-limiting effects. In the case of Lucy, a cycle has emerged in which she adopts ever more vigilant safety behaviours to avoid vomiting or being in the presence of a person who is vomiting. However, her fear remains undiminished as she has failed to become habituated herself to the original fear of vomit or vomiting.

4 **What therapeutic interventions might help Lucy?**

A Despite the prevalence of phobia among the population because it is a related condition, guidance for the treatment of phobia is listed alongside the recommended treatments for the range of anxiety disorders (NCCMH 2011).

Medication is generally only considered necessary to reduce the symptoms of anxiety which accompany phobias. Instead psychological therapies are generally favoured. These can take the form of the following treatments:

- support groups;
- counselling;
- self-help literature (available from local libraries, GP surgeries and other healthcare professionals);
- support from family, peers and friends;
- computerized cognitive behavioural therapy (CCBT);
- cognitive behavioural therapy (CBT), which is the case for Lucy.

A CBT approach which has been recommended for phobia is to confront the source of the fear through **exposure**, and commonly this takes the form of **graded exposure** (Emmelkemp 2004). However, confronting the fear is contrary to most people's response which instead involves safety behaviours or defence mechanisms to prevent their encountering the feared phenomena. Therefore, most people with phobias go untreated, often preferring to live with the fear rather than confront it due to the extreme anxiety and distress which this might provoke (Veale 2009).

Due to the feelings of vulnerability and significant anxiety that people with phobias such as Lucy experience, exposure needs to be implemented sensitively and within a supportive and collaborative therapeutic relationship which actively empowers the person. Although CBT is a time-limited treatment, the therapist met Lucy a number of times to establish a trusting and working rapport. Lucy's motivation to overcome her fear was her deeply felt wish to start a family. However, she was still terrified about what the treatment might involve, and made it clear that she needed to feel as though she were in control.

A chronological history was taken of Lucy's experiences of vomiting from her earliest memories (Veale 2009). Although the event which triggered her phobia occurred more than 20 years ago, Lucy still experienced a clear recollection of the event in the form of a flashback which had a very powerful impact on her feelings. Lucy had found the sight, sound and smell profoundly shocking and repellent and retained a very vivid image in her memory. At the time of the event, Lucy felt nauseous and feared that she might also vomit. She thought that being sick in front of others might traumatize them and she would also find it devastatingly shameful. This suggests that Lucy identified with the boy she witnessed vomiting, and was unable to separate the notion of witnessing vomiting from being sick herself.

During the discussion with the therapist, it was evident that Lucy was unable to tolerate use of the word 'vomit', preferring the term 'it', while she also spoke in very vague terms about the problem in order to avoid her description triggering the anxiety-provoking images. Lucy said that she was concerned that talking to the therapist about vomiting might lead her to be sick. The therapist asked Lucy what she felt would be the worst outcome and she replied that she might vomit and the therapist would be disgusted.

The therapist then asked Lucy where she might safely vomit, if this were the case and Lucy identified a wastepaper basket. The wastepaper basket was placed close to Lucy during the session. Often people with fears or phobias make catastrophic predictions of events which might happen. By building in a safety mechanism in the event of the worst case scenario, the therapist was supporting Lucy by providing a plan.

When working collaboratively with the person in appraising their fears, it helps to be able to quantify them. In CBT this is most commonly achieved by asking the person to rate their fear or anxiety. The therapist therefore asked Lucy to rate her fear of vomit or vomiting when using the word 'vomit' on a scale of 1–10, with 1 being the lowest. Lucy rated her fear at 10. This has the therapeutic effect of allowing the person to reflect on their feelings rather than being unquestioningly compelled by them. Often feelings of fear are experienced as impulses which the person feels unable to control. However, if the person assesses the strength of the fear, they can begin to question this response and whether this is proportionate to the stimuli which cause it to occur.

However, scoring her fears was also central to the process by which Lucy would be involved with graded exposure. The therapist discussed with Lucy that they might develop a **hierarchy of fears** together and compile a list of phenomena pertaining to Lucy's fear of vomit or vomiting. They would then rate them in relation to the level of fear which they triggered in her and then agree for her to be exposed to certain selected experiences.

Through overcoming her fears by using these staged intervals it was intended that Lucy would develop **habituation** to vomit and vomiting and gain in confidence and that her fear would reduce. However, the successive stages of progression through the hierarchy were carefully negotiated between Lucy and the therapist so that Lucy felt in control.

Lucy then agreed to carry out a behavioural experiment and say the word 'vomit' aloud, repeatedly, and after each time rate her anxiety out of 10 until it no longer provoked an anxious or fear reaction. To Lucy's surprise, this only took about 10 minutes. Following discussion with the therapist and confident from her success, Lucy then engaged in another behavioural experiment, practising writing the word while saying it aloud and again rating her anxiety until it subsided.

Following these behavioural experiments, Lucy discussed with the therapist what she had learned. Lucy identified that she had been able to tolerate both the word 'vomit' and the related anxiety it caused without vomiting and that over time the anxiety subsided. The learning for her was that confronting the word 'vomit' and the images which she associated with it was helpful in the longer term.

Next, Lucy and the therapist identified a series of most feared and avoided situations regarding vomit and vomiting and placed them in the order that would cause her least distress up to the most. It is important that the person makes the choice of the item on which to work rather than addressing them in their order on the hierarchy from the least to most anxiety-provoking. Lucy chose an item from near the bottom of the hierarchy and which was less of a challenge to work on in the next session, which was looking at black and white pictures of vomit.

The therapist brought along a number of black and white pictures of vomit to the next section which Lucy graded in order of awfulness. From the least to most anxiety-provoking, the images included vomit in a bowl, vomit in a sink, vomit in a toilet, vomit on the floor, and finally vomit on a person.

Lucy began by looking at the pictures one after another in a drawer with the least awful first, and then they were brought out of the drawer one at a time with Lucy's permission. The pictures were not turned over until she agreed. Initially Lucy stood at a distance from the pictures and gradually moved nearer to the picture as she felt able to until her anxiety diminished and she could tolerate turning over, holding and touching the picture.

In discussion with the therapist at the end of the session, Lucy identified that her learning was that the longer she avoided and prolonged turning the pictures over, the more anxious she became, whereas the quicker she turned over the picture, the more rapidly her anxiety subsided. This was not what she had expected but it significantly influenced her approach to therapy in future weeks. Lucy took the pictures home and kept looking at them throughout the week as agreed homework.

Therapy progressed through the hierarchy of exposure which Lucy had agreed with the therapist, progressing to coloured pictures of vomit, then to clips of people vomiting, which were played repeatedly, first with the sound down and then including sound, until her anxiety subsided. Such interventions have been found to be effective in fears of vomit and vomiting.

As agreed homework between sessions, Lucy also went to places which she would normally avoid to test whether her fears were proven correct. On one occasion a man in a nightclub did vomit in the foyer and she was surprised that she was able to make herself go toward rather than avoid the area where this occurred.

Finally, Lucy was exposed to some fake vomit. Lucy was aware that the vomit was not real but it was made from a recipe which closely simulated this substance of porridge oats, tomato, and carrot and parmesan cheese. The fake vomit was initially placed in a urine specimen bottle labelled 'vomit'. Once Lucy felt able, she could pick this up and shake it about in a session with a minimum of anxiety, and she was encouraged to put it into her bag to carry around for the week as homework.

Lucy's most feared outcome, despite repeatedly examining the specimen bottle in the session and finding it to be both robust and secure, was that it would leak or break in her bag. A plan was devised in case this should occur, Lucy would put her bag inside two plastic bags which she would keep with her and she would bring it to the therapist at the next session.

The final exposure involved Lucy emptying the contents of the specimen bottle into the sink and clearing the sink. She thought that if she could manage this, she would have overcome her fear of vomit. Lucy successfully achieved this goal and stated how good she felt about herself and that she now felt ready to try for a baby.

CONCLUSION

Many people experience phobias; however, they prefer to live with the fear rather than undergo the anxiety involved with exposure. Lucy had significant motivation for wanting to address her phobia which provided her with the resolve to overcome her fears. It is important when working with people who have phobias to appreciate the level of anxiety involved, to work at their pace and to fully involve the person collaboratively to make decisions on the goals and activities to undertake. In Lucy's case, the therapist implemented the therapeutic approach of graded exposure, yet central to success was carefully developing a fully collaborative and trusting therapeutic relationship.

REFERENCES

Emmelkemp, P.M.G. (2004) Behaviour therapy with adults, in M.J. Lambert (ed.) *Bergin and Garfield's Handbook of Psychotherapy and Behaviour Change*, 5th edn. Chicago: John Wiley and Sons, Inc., pp. 393–446.

NCCMH (National Collaborating Centre for Mental Health) (2011) National Clinical Guideline Number 123, *Common Mental Health Disorders: Identification and Pathways to Care*. London: NICE.

NHS Choices (2011) *Phobias*. Available at: http://www.nhs.uk/conditions/Phobias/Pages/Introduction. aspx (accessed 30 September 2011).

Veale, D. (2009) Cognitive behaviour therapy for a specific phobia of vomiting, *The Cognitive Behaviour Therapist* 2: 272–88.

FURTHER RESOURCES FOR PEOPLE WITH EMETOPHOBIA

Anxiety UK (formerly National Phobics Society)
Zion Community Resource Centre,
339 Stretford Road,
Hulme,
Manchester M15 4ZY
Tel.: 08444 775 774
http://www.anxietyuk.org.uk

Dental Anxiety and Phobia Association
104 Harley Street,
London W1G 7JD
Tel.: 020 7935 8092
http://www.healthyteeth.com

Gut Reaction
PO Box 70,
Ross-on-Wye,
Herefordshire HR9 5YP
http://www.gut-reaction.freeserve.co.uk

NO PANIC (National Organisation for Phobias, Anxiety, Neuroses, Information and Care)
93 Brands Farm Way,
Randley,
Telford,
Shropshire TF3 2JQ
Helpline: 0808 808 0545
http://www.nopanic.org.uk

Triumph Over Phobia (TOP UK)
PO Box 3760,
Bath BA2 3WY
Tel.: 0845 600 9601
http://www.triumphoverphobia.com

Runs a national network of structured, self-help groups for adults (16+) suffering from phobias.

CASE STUDY 11
Post-traumatic stress disorder (PTSD)
Nick Wrycraft and Noel Sawyer

Sue is 42 and married with two teenage children. She has experienced low mood intermittently for the past ten years, and she takes anti-depressant medication for this. Recently Sue's
mental health has become worse after being bullied by her manager at work, and experiencing
marital difficulties at home. Her G P increased her prescription, but Sue found it made her
sleepy and produced side effects.

Due to her low mood, Sue has been signed off from work for the past three months.
Although her G P has suggested being referred to the specialist mental health services several
times before, Sue has always resisted. However, in discussion with her G P, Sue reluctantly
agreed to be referred to a therapist trained in cognitive behavioural therapy (CBT) who
liaises with the surgery.

Sue attended an assessment with the therapist and was anxious and very low in mood,
avoiding eye contact and lacking animation in her expression. Sue said that she felt guilty for
not coping with her responsibilities at home, that her concentration and memory were poor
and she had reduced motivation and energy. Since being off sick from work, Sue has become
reluctant to leave the house, avoiding contact with people whenever possible. She wakes up
early each morning and comfort eats throughout the day. Sue often stays in bed all day in an
attempt to block out intrusive thoughts. Sue has also stopped caring for herself and washing.
She is also often troubled by the thought of abuse happening to her children and of her being
unable to protect them.

During the assessment the therapist asked more about Sue's background. She describes not
remembering much of her early life but what she can recall are memories of being neglected,
often left alone and being uncared for and abused. Sue's mother was verbally and physically
aggressive, often criticizing and shouting at her, while easily losing her temper and she was
frequently hit and beaten for little or no reason. Sue's dad was often absent and, when he was
at home, displayed no interest in her. She often went to school unwashed and in dirty clothes
and was teased by other children. Sue later experienced sexual abuse in her teens and although
she has never spoken about this, it has left her feeling highly vulnerable and a deep-seated
sense of shame and self-loathing. The lower in mood and fatigued Sue has become, the more
focused she has become on threat and failure.

In spite of these difficulties Sue was outwardly sociable and established a wide social
network and left school with good qualifications. Sue has always worked and has been married
for 18 years and always been an active person. However, she always regarded herself as a
failure, and considered other people and the world at large as being unsafe and untrustworthy.
While having a number of friends, these were superficial relationships. Sue was very vigilant
of others and anxious not to be taken advantage of and avoided talking about her feelings and
revealing too much about herself. She thoroughly planned all aspects of her life to ensure that

things did not go wrong and she did not lose control of situations. For example, Sue often made all of the arrangements for social gatherings and would lock outside doors at home or at work if she was alone in the building. Sue was also keen to please others and always avoided any difficult situation or conflict whenever possible.

However, several relationships failed and Sue came to believe that in some cases people sensed her vulnerability and deliberately took advantage of her or placed her in compromising situations. Recently a colleague at work was promoted as her manager and began to make increasing demands of her and criticize her, which undermined Sue's confidence, yet Sue felt unable to confront this colleague. At the same time she has become more distant from her husband, leading to frequent arguments and relationship problems. Recently Sue admitted that she took an overdose of tablets in an attempt to end her life.

In accordance with CBT practice the therapist identified a case formulation for Sue (Figure 11.1). The lack of safe attachment figures in her early life meant that Sue saw herself as a failure and other people and the world in general as unsafe and untrustworthy. Her later experience of sexual abuse resulted in an intensification of feelings of vulnerability and a lack of safety while reinforcing her **core beliefs** of seeing herself as a failure.

Sue's response was to seek to form amicable relationships with other people and to please them and avoid conflict but remain vigilant and avoid investing too much in social relationships, plan her life to excess, and make sure that things did not go wrong. However, the relationship failures added further confirmation to her negative feelings about herself and loss of confidence in her coping mechanisms. Sue responded by isolating herself, remaining in bed, not washing and avoiding leaving the house. Her self-neglect reminded her of her childhood which undermined her attempts to block the intrusive thoughts. As Sue's mood has become lower, her negative feelings have increased and she has felt trapped and unable to cope, leading to suicidal thoughts and a serious attempt at suicide.

1   What is post-traumatic stress disorder (PTSD)?

A   Post-traumatic stress disorder (PTSD) can result from traumatic and distressing life experiences (NHS Choices 2009). In children, it can occur as a result of abuse and or neglect. In adulthood, PTSD can be caused by severe and repeated violence or abuse. For example:

- experiences in situations of war;
- torture or abusive imprisonment;
- rape, sexual and emotional abuse;
- difficult childbirth;
- witnessing violent death or injury/mutilation;
- other situations where the person felt extremely distressed, their life was endangered and they were helpless.

(NICE 2005; NHS Choices 2009; Royal College of Psychiatrists 2010)

PTSD was first identified in combat veterans, and characteristic of this mental health problem is that it is a response to experiencing traumatic, violent or aggressive events. It is not triggered by anxiety-provoking events such as losing a job, failing an exam or divorce, although these can still be stressful experiences which cause high levels of anxiety (NHS Choices 2009).

PTSD can occur where feelings we take for granted of being safe and secure are suddenly undermined, and we are made aware of our own mortality (RCP 2010). Many people will

Early Experiences

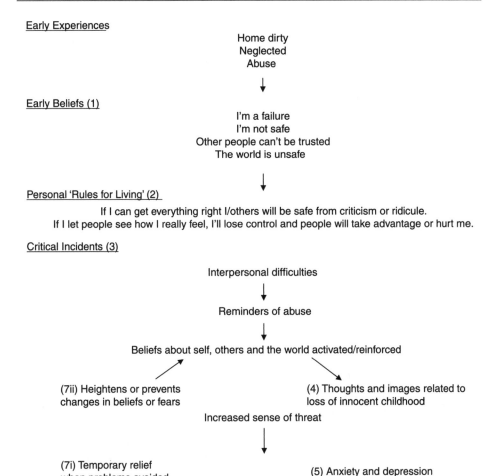

Home dirty
Neglected
Abuse

↓

Early Beliefs (1)

I'm a failure
I'm not safe
Other people can't be trusted
The world is unsafe

↓

Personal 'Rules for Living' (2)

If I can get everything right I/others will be safe from criticism or ridicule.
If I let people see how I really feel, I'll lose control and people will take advantage or hurt me.

Critical Incidents (3)

Interpersonal difficulties

↓

Reminders of abuse

↓

Beliefs about self, others and the world activated/reinforced

(7ii) Heightens or prevents
changes in beliefs or fears

(4) Thoughts and images related to
loss of innocent childhood

Increased sense of threat

↓

(7i) Temporary relief
when problems avoided

(5) Anxiety and depression

(6) Safety Behaviours

Hypervigilance
Protection of children
Perfectionism, people pleasing, appearing confident

↓

Escape and avoidance
Not expressing emotions

↓

Staying in bed
Suicide attempts

Figure 11.1 Sue's case formulation

Note: Anxiety and depression have been placed in the same domain to illustrate how easily one may lead to the other. At times, either emotion could override the other's safety behaviour. For example, her need to escape from sad thoughts led her to neglect housework and remain in bed although thoughts of her daughter walking home from school alone were enough to make her get up and go and collect her.

experience a brief and time-limited stress-related response following traumatic experiences which dissipates within a few weeks, however, around 30 per cent of people who experience a traumatic event will develop PTSD (NHS Choices 2009). PTSD can occur some time or even many years after the traumatic experience.

Common factors which can prolong PTSD include:

- where the traumatic events occur suddenly and unexpectedly;
- where the traumatic events occur over a sustained period of time;
- where the person is unable to avoid the events;
- where there are many deaths;
- where there is significant mutilation, for example, the loss of limbs;
- where children are involved.

(RCP 2010)

In addition to emotional responses such as grief, anxiety, guilt or anger, the person might experience three main features in PTSD. These are:

- **Flashbacks** *and nightmares* – where the person repeatedly relives the traumatic event either in the daytime or in dreams and this can be experienced as a very vivid and realistic experience. Features of everyday life which resemble aspects of the experience can be sufficient to trigger off flashbacks; for example, if a person has been in a battlefield conflict in which there was loud gunfire, the sound of a car backfiring might lead to their reliving this experience (NICE 2005; RCP 2010; NCCMH 2011).
- **Avoidance** *and* **numbing** – the experience of reliving the memories may be too distressing, leading to the person engaging in distracting activities. These may take the form of recreational activities, hobbies and leisure interests. However, another form of coping is for the person not to engage emotionally and numb their feelings (RCP 2010). They may withdraw from contact with other people and feel isolated, detached and emotionally numb (NHS Choices 2009; NCCMH 2011). Alternatively the person may use food, drugs, or alcohol as a means of blocking out intrusive traumatic thoughts or feelings.
- Hypervigilance – The person will be excessively watchful of their surroundings and of others to the extent of not sleeping and being suspicious of others and constantly anxious (RCP 2010).

PTSD often goes unrecognized due to many of the features of this problem resembling, and being experienced co-morbidly with depression and anxiety. It is estimated that between 80–90 per cent of people with PTSD will experience other mental health problems such as depression and anxiety (NICE 2005). Another feature of this mental health problem is that the person attempts to avoid or has impaired recollection of the distressing memories and may not wish to discuss the source of their trauma.

2   **Which features of Sue's case are consistent with PTSD?**

   - Sue has experienced childhood physical, psychological and sexual abuse, all of which are identified as triggers for PTSD.
- Sue describes not remembering much about her early life and does not discuss the sexual abuse which she experienced. Both of these factors are consistent with avoidance

and numbing, as she does not want to relive the distress associated with these experiences.

- Often in childhood and sexual abuse, the victim is unable to exert any power to avoid it occurring, which can worsen the traumatic effects.
- Sue is very vigilant of others in her social relationships and avoids revealing personal information.
- Sue wakes up early in the morning which is linked with hypervigilance.
- Sue appears to be experiencing flashbacks in the form of recurring intrusive thoughts.
- Sue is engaging in comfort eating to avoid her intrusive thoughts.
- Although Sue has coped for many years, her experiencing PTSD now is consistent with how people sometimes experience this problem.

3 **What treatments might help with PTSD?**

A The first line of treatment which is recommended for PTSD is trauma-focused psychological therapy which emphasizes the use of imagery (NICE 2005). Medication such as anti-depressants is not recommended for PTSD, but will help with the physical features and aspects of PTSD related to depression and anxiety (NICE 2005; RCP 2010). The only drug licensed for use with PTSD in the UK is **paroxetine** (NCCMH 2011).

Sue clearly presented a high level of risk and the therapist discussed with her that she might need an in-patient admission. Sue was reluctant to agree to this; however, the therapist reassessed Sue's risk in each session.

Sue was reluctant to talk about her past in therapy, finding it distressing to contemplate. The therapist agreed with this, and often when working with people with PTSD, the focus in the initial stages of therapy is on other symptoms. Therefore, even though she is experiencing PTSD, her work with the therapist focused on Sue's current experience of depression.

4 **What rationales support this approach?**

A
- It is important that the person sets the goals in therapy in order for these to have personal meaning.
- Sue's long-standing strategy in relationships is to avoid divulging personal information through feeling vulnerable. It is only reasonable to expect her to need time to develop a rapport with the therapist sufficient for her to feel safe.
- Improving Sue's mood first will better prepare her to cope with her deeper-rooted feelings in time, should she feel able.
- It is advisable to avoid addressing deep-rooted problems early in therapy as this will worsen the person's mood and potentially further undermine Sue's mental state when she already feels a significant degree of hopelessness and has attempted suicide.

The therapist worked with Sue for over 50 sessions, which is consistent with other similar cases where progress is time-consuming with the person needing to learn new ways of inter-acting with others, challenge ingrained beliefs and develop new ones (Lee 2005).

The goals which the therapist and Sue agreed and worked on were as follows:

- In the beginning, Sue was reluctant to engage in therapy, but did accept that it might work. Also all her life, Sue has been skilled in establishing social relationships which were superficial as she is cautious in revealing information about herself through suspicion of others. It was therefore important to focus on establishing a trusting therapeutic rapport with the therapist to avoid replicating these previous relationships which she had invested in to only a limited extent.

- Through collaboration with the therapist, Sue agreed that she wanted to increase her activity by using a schedule. The purpose of the activity schedule was to help structure her day, and to plan and increase the actions she undertook (BBC n.d.) (see Table 8.1 on p. 68). This would draw to her attention data that would support the belief that she was coping and therefore was not a failure.
- Sue also re-evaluated her negative thoughts by using thought records (Table 11.1). These helped her re-evaluate her negative self-appraisals. Sue found that the thought records helped her to maintain a sense of balance in her thinking.

During the course of her therapy the use of the activity records and thought records relieved Sue's feelings of pervasive low mood and her mental health overall improved. However, at times when she was low, her core feelings of being a failure, distrusting others and feeling vulnerable re-emerged and Sue developed concerns about relapsing.

In discussion with the therapist, Sue was encouraged to recognize that when her emotions were low, the rational evaluation and understanding which she had developed that she was not a failure were dismissed, and instead her feelings rejected this appraisal. Ingrained and deep-rooted feelings are often difficult for people to challenge, even where there is evidence to the contrary and Sue's feeling that she was a failure represented a **schema**, or core belief.

In discussion with Sue about tackling her core belief of being a failure, the therapist suggested working on a data log to attempt to balance this belief by considering other beliefs which she might have. In agreeing what an alternative belief might be, Sue felt that the reverse belief that she was successful was too far from her current belief to be obtainable, and so she agreed on the belief that she can cope. As her confidence in her ability to cope

Table 11.1 Example of a thought record

Situation	Moods	Automatic thought	Evidence	Evidence	Alternative/ balanced thoughts	Mood rating
The moment when the bad feelings began	How we feel, for example, angry, sad or anxious	Identify the 'hot' thought most closely associated with negative feelings	Consider the negative evidence	Consider the positive evidence	Return to the thought and restate it in the light of the evidence in columns 4 and 5	Rate the thought in column 2 again to see the effect of the thought record

developed, the therapist took it a step further and Sue began to record instances of her being capable and eventually competent.

As Sue's confidence began to grow, she began to do things differently and break some of her established patterns of behaviour, for example, by beginning to talk a little about her early life experiences. Such work resulted in a series of behavioural experiments conducted to test possible alternative outcomes in her 'natural world'. These experiments were linked to a 'Historical Log' of significant times in the past when she had not abided by her strict personal rules and her feared consequences had not occurred. Such data was recorded and used in discussions during therapy sessions.

The final phase of therapy focused on developing self-compassion rather than self-criticism and blame. This was particularly difficult for Sue as compassion and caring were unfamiliar and frightening and she associated this state with being vulnerable. Sue eventually found the technique used of writing comforting letters as being helpful. She also reflected on other strategies she had learned and began a **comforting data log**, regularly doing and recording comforting things for herself. This work is ongoing although the outcome looks promising.

By the end of the CBT sessions, Sue's mood and anxiety had improved and the frequency and intensity with which she experienced intrusive thoughts had significantly reduced. Sue's marital relationship was better and she had returned to work and was considering her future career. By providing a regular, reliable and consistent contact and by the collaborative use of various treatment strategies, the therapist was able to effectively contain Sue's distress. This seemed to provide Sue with useful stability and was reinforced by developing confidence in her ability to address and modify her negative schemas. Sue was better able to see her own abilities, and re-evaluate her negative thoughts. The degree of improvement in Sue's core beliefs and assumptions was significant and would help protect her from further depression, although it should be noted that negative beliefs may be re-activated at times of future stress. Continued practice and reflection are required to maintain progress. This was understandably difficult, given her lifelong self-criticism but, like previous strategies, improved with continued practice.

REFERENCES

BBC (n. d.) Activity scheduling: the fabulous four, in *Headroom Well-being Guide*. Available at: http://downloads.bbc.co.uk/headroom/cbt/activity_scheduling.pdf (accessed 25 October 2011).

Lee, D.A. (2005) The perfect nurturer: A model to develop compassion within cognitive therapy, in P. Gilbert (ed.) *Compassion and Psychotherapy: Theory, Research and Practice*. London: Routledge.

NCCMH (National Collaborating Centre for Mental Health) (2011) National Clinical Guideline Number 123, *Common Mental Health Disorders: Identification and Pathways to Care*. London: NICE.

NHS Choices (2009) *Post-traumatic stress disorder*. Available at: http://www.nhs.uk/Conditions/Post-traumatic-stress-disorder/Pages/Introduction.aspx (accessed 11 October 2011).

NICE (National Institute for Health and Clinical Excellence) (2005) *Post-Traumatic Stress Disorder (PTSD): The Treatment of PTSD in Adults and Children: Understanding NICE Guidance – Information for People with PTSD, Their Advocates and Carers, and the Public*. Available at: http://www.nice.org.uk/nicemedia/pdf/CG026publicinfo.pdf (accessed 11 October 2011).

RCP (Royal College of Psychiatrists) (2010) *Post Traumatic Stress Disorder*. Available at: http://www.rcpsych.ac.uk/mentalhealthinfo/problems/ptsd/posttraumaticstressdisorder.aspx (accessed 9 October 2011).

FURTHER READING

American Psychiatric Association (2000) *Diagnostic and Statistical Manual of Mental Disorders*, 4th edn, text revision. Washington, DC: APA.

Beck, A.T. (1996) Beyond belief: a theory of modes, personality and psychopathology, in P. M. Salkovskis (ed.) *Frontiers of Cognitive Therapy*. New York: Guilford Press.

Beck, A.T., Rush, A.J., Shaw, B.F. and Emery, G. (1979) *Cognitive Therapy of Depression*. New York: Guilford Press.

Chard, K.M., Weaver, T.L. and Resick, P.A. (1997) Adapting cognitive processing therapy for child sexual abuse survivors, *Cognitive and Behavioural Practice*, 4: 31–52.

Clark, D.A. and Steer, R.A. (1996) Empirical status of the cognitive model of anxiety and depression, in P. M. Salkovskis (ed.) *Frontiers of Cognitive Therapy*. New York: Guilford Press.

Ehlers, A. and Clark, D. M. (2000) A cognitive model of posttraumatic stress disorder, *Behaviour Research and Therapy*, 38: 319–45.

Gilbert, P. (2007) *Psychotherapy and Counselling for Depression*, 3rd edn. London: Sage.

Resick, P.A. and Schnicke, M.K. (1992) Cognitive processing therapy for sexual assault victims, *Journal of Consulting and Clinical Psychology*, 60: 748–56.

Thwaites, R. and Freeston, M.H. (2005) Safety-seeking behaviours: fact or function – how can we clinically differentiate between safety behaviours and adaptive coping strategies across anxiety disorders? *Behavioural and Cognitive Psychotherapy*, 33: 177–88.

Van der Kolk, B.A., Roth, S., Pelcovitz, D. and Sunday, S. (2005) Disorders of extreme stress: the empirical foundation of a complex adaptation to trauma, *Journal of Traumatic Stress*, 18(5): 389–99.

Williams, J.M.G., Thorsten, B., Crane, C. and Beck, A.T. (2005) Problem solving deteriorates following mood challenge in formerly depressed patients with a history of suicidal ideation, *Journal of Abnormal Psychology*, 114(3): 421–31.

PART 3
Other Types of Mental Health Problems in Adults

CASE STUDY 12
Alcohol misuse
Nick Wrycraft

Mary is 32 years old and has attended the Accident and Emergency (A & E) department accompanied by her long-term partner Martin after falling down some stairs in her home. On three occasions recently she has visited A & E, having sustained injuries while under the influence of alcohol. On each occasion she has been referred for a mental health liaison appointment with a nurse based at A & E to discuss her drinking once the effects of the alcohol have subsided.

Mary has had a considerable wait at the hospital, has received treatment, is medically fit and can go home, but just needs to speak with the mental health nurse concerning her alcohol usage. She seems restless, and keen to leave, not seeing the necessity of discussing her alcohol use, as she does not believe she has a problem. Mary looks dishevelled in appearance and her breath smells of alcohol. Her eyes appear red and she is complaining of a headache and needing to drink water frequently.

1   **What do you understand to be the psychological and physical effects of alcohol?**

A   *Psychologically* alcohol brings about chemical changes which affect the brain and mood, emotion and behaviour and can lead people to behave differently. Examples include the loss of inhibitions, aggression, and tearfulness or excessive humour. Other effects include rapid changes in mood with poor or impulsive decision making and behaviour. Alcohol is also linked to mood disorders, depression, anxiety and even psychosis (Drinkaware 2010a).

Prolonged alcohol misuse has been linked with various psychological problems including memory damage and impaired brain functioning (Drinkaware 2010b), while Korsakoff's syndrome is a form of dementia frequently experienced specifically due to alcohol misuse. Other dementia-type illnesses, such as vascular dementia and small vessel disease, are also more likely (Drinkaware 2010a).

In the short term, Mary might feel that there are few, if any, consequences for her. However, the common instant *physical* effects of alcohol even in moderation are to impair coordination and reflexes, leading to accidents, such as Mary has been experiencing. Alcohol is a toxin which the body works hard to process, placing stress on the liver and kidneys and leading to dehydration and effects such as hangovers. The consequences of sustained alcohol misuse include a wide range of problems, including kidney and liver damage, cirrhosis, nerve damage, high blood pressure (hypertension), diabetes, heart problems and duodenal, oesophageal and throat cancer. For women of child-bearing age such as Mary, foetal alcohol syndrome (FAS) and damage to the unborn child are a risk (Drinkaware 2010a).

Mary is reluctant to speak with us, and so before we can assess her use of alcohol we need to carefully consider how to engage with her, using both verbal and non-verbal communication. Using verbal communication: after introducing ourselves, we ask whether Mary agrees for Martin to be present for the discussion.

2   **How might we begin a conversation with Mary?**

A   Although we already have some information, Mary is the expert on her own experience, and so asking Mary what has happened in her own words is helpful. Using **open questions**, for example, 'Can you tell me about what happened to you today?' and allowing the person to provide their own answer, as opposed to **closed questions**, which require a 'yes' or 'no' answer will encourage Mary to speak to us.

Using non-verbal communication: although what we say is important, our non-verbal communication creates a much greater impression.

3   **What kind of non-verbal communication can we use with Mary to create a positive impression?**

A   Retaining appropriate eye contact, being friendly and using **active listening**, for example nodding at intervals and responding with positive facial gestures which match and respond to what Mary says.

Using **unconditional positive regard** is important (Rogers 1983). Developing an effective therapeutic relationship involves actively demonstrating positive and non-judgemental attitudes in our verbal and non-verbal communication, and to see the world through the person's eyes while avoiding imposing our own values and views, for example, not giving our opinions or views in response to what Mary tells us, but instead actively listening and being positive in communicating with Mary.

A range of different assessment tools are used in clinical practice from CAGE (Ewing 1984) to AUDIT, AUDIT-PC, AUDIT-C, FAST and SASQ (Newcastle University 2006); however, no single set of questions is universally applicable, and while Trusts and teams often have standardized assessment tools as part of their protocols, these can still be used discreetly highlighting the aspects which are relevant. Asking a person about behaviours which clearly do not apply to them, such as how much they drink socially when it is well established that the nature of their alcohol misuse is their drinking alone is best avoided, although assessments need to gather a wide range of information which may reveal issues we did not expect, or even might differ from what the person themselves regards as the problem. It is also best to be careful and sensitive in asking questions which the person may feel to be highly negative as this can damage the therapeutic relationship, especially at the very preliminary stage as we are at with Mary. Assessment needs to be flexible and centred around further developing the therapeutic rapport with Mary and fostering her engagement and trust.

Table 12.1 shows a selection of questions from some of the above-mentioned tools, indicating the range of areas of a person's functioning which are frequently affected by the misuse use of alcohol. The government has also issued specific guidance on harmful and **safe drinking levels** which is useful for assessing cases where alcohol is the biggest problem but also in the case of other people where alcohol misuse is part of a multi-faceted problem (DoH 2007; NICE 2010).

Martin is concerned that Mary's alcohol consumption is 'out of control', saying that she drinks heavily on a daily basis and he feels she is physically and psychologically dependent and cannot just have one drink but instead drinks compulsively. Martin says Mary has lied about her alcohol intake and has hidden alcohol in the home. Martin says that Mary's mother had a long-term alcohol problem, and suggests that her behaviour is beginning to resemble this pattern.

Table 12.1 Useful questions in assessing drinking behaviour

How often in the last year have you found you were not able to stop drinking once you had started?

How often have you failed to do what was expected of you because of your drinking?

How often in the last year have you had a feeling of guilt or regret after drinking?

How often in the last year have you not been able to remember what happened after drinking the night before?

How often do you drink alone?

Have you, or someone else been injured as a result of your drinking?

In the last year, have you been in trouble as a result of your drinking?

Has a relative/friend/doctor/health worker been concerned about your drinking, or advised you to cut down?

Have you experienced hangovers which prevented you from attending work or being able to carry out pre-planned activities?

Have you needed to have a drink to reduce feelings of craving or anxiety?

How often in the last year have you drunk first thing in the morning?

Source: Newcastle University (2006).

Table 12.2 Guidelines for safe drinking

	Maximum units per day	Maximum units per week	Increased risk drinking (per week)	Higher risk drinking (per week)
Adult men	3–4 units	21 units	22–50 units	50 units+
Adult women	2–3 units	14 units	15–35 units	35 units+
Pregnant women or women trying for a baby	1–2 units once or twice per week			

Notes: A unit of alcohol is 8g or 10ml of ethanol (DoH 2007; NICE 2010). It is also recommended that anyone consuming a large amount of alcohol in one session abstain from drinking for the next 48 hours to allow their liver and body tissue time to repair.

4 **Which of the above factors might be features of an alcohol problem?**

A All of the above. Drinking on a daily basis can indicate **alcohol dependence**, which can be physical, psychological or both. Alcoholics Anonymous (2010) define **problem drinking** as where the person experiences a compulsion to drink beyond their control. People often under-report the amount they have drunk either knowingly out of embarrassment or through simply having no recollection, and may hide alcohol due to the strength of their attachment and needing to have access to a supply. It is also often the case that people with an alcohol problem have relatives who themselves misused alcohol.

Mary now begins to talk more openly, and states that she is employed in a professional job with a high profile firm and has worked with the same company now for a number of years, progressing very well. Her job is very stressful and involves a high level of responsibility and socializing with clients and contacts. Throughout her life she describes herself as having very high expectations of herself and being a perfectionist.

Yet Mary still shrugs off any suggestion that she has a problem with alcohol, saying that she likes to drink and does it to unwind, and many of her colleagues drink heavily as well. She quotes a recent article in the media stating that many professional people drink to alleviate stress yet still perform to a high level.

Alcohol is sometimes used as a coping mechanism in stressful and high pressured jobs, and also where people have perfectionist or high personal expectations (BBC 2010). The social acceptability and availability of alcohol can lead people to either disguise or deny they have a problem, while people with a latent tendency may gradually develop a problem due to their lifestyle. Furthermore, there is a powerful social stigma stereotyping people who misuse alcohol as profligate and undesirable, leading to people with alcohol problems feeling a deep sense of shame (NCCMH 2011). The contrast between Martin and Mary's perception illustrates how in close relationships partners or significant others often identify the problem before the person themselves, which can cause friction.

THE STAGES OF CHANGE MODEL

Changing behaviour can be difficult and requires significant motivation and effort on the part of the person if it is to be successful. To be able to work effectively with Mary and make progress, it is necessary to establish the extent of her motivation to change. The **stages of change model** of Prochaska and DiClemente (1986) is a five-stage model, often used with people who have addiction issues, and works on the premise that successful behaviour change occurs in stages and progress will be at different rates for different people (AddictionInfo.org 2010) (Table 12.3).

Often people who reach the action stage experience relapse, which is the sixth stage of the model. The final stage of the model has been identified as transcendence, which occurs where the maintenance stage has endured for sufficiently long to allow the person to be able to reflect on their previous behaviour and regard it in a new light as it no longer is a central part of their life.

5   **Which of the stages of change model do you believe would apply to Mary?**

A   Mary seems to be at the pre-contemplation stage, as she does not accept there is a problem and defends her drinking behaviour. However, part of her argument is that many of her colleagues drink heavily as well, indicating that she accepts that she drinks heavily which demonstrates some insight on her behaviour, so she may be at the pre-contemplation stage of the model.

People do not always move forward through the stages of the model at an even rate, and as is the case with Mary it is not unusual for a person to be between stages at the same time or even go back stages. However, it is important to avoid losing hope but to persevere in the understanding that change is possible even when repeated attempts to change have ended in relapse (AddictionInfo.org 2010).

Martin says that he is concerned that as Mary's drinking has increased after recent problems at work, it will be harder for her to stop. He does not go on to identify what these were, instead indicating to her that Mary ought to explain.

Table 12.3 The stages of change model

Stage of the model	Explanation	Characteristics of a person at this stage
Pre-contemplation	Does not accept that there is a problem	The person is not interested in help which might be available and are likely to even defend their current behaviour
Contemplation	Aware of the problem, but not yet ready to act	The person is aware of the harmful consequences of their behaviour. The person may well have balanced up the negatives and positives of their behaviour but require more convincing that the positives outweigh the negatives in the longer term
Preparation/ Determination	Commitment to change	Small steps have been made towards changing the harmful behaviour, for example, gathering information about what needs to be carried out in order to change
Action/Willpower	Steps are taken to change behaviour	The shortest of the stages but can still last for between 6 months to 6 hours or briefer and relies on willpower. Short-term rewards may be used to retain motivation and appreciating small successes is necessary. In this stage the person is most likely to be receptive to help and assistance
Maintenance	Continued change of behaviour and avoidance of returning to previous behaviour	Successful avoidance of returning to previous behavioural pattern. In this stage the person has acquired new coping skills and strategies and identified methods of dealing with avoiding the temptation to revert to old behaviours

Source: Adapted from AddictionInfo.org (2010).

Mary seems more willing to confide now, and says that she was turned down for a promotion she was sure she would get. Since then Mary has been having doubts about her career, feels resentful towards her employers for not gaining the promotion, and believes that she was overlooked because she is a woman.

6 **Does Mary's increased drinking make changing her behaviour more difficult than it was before?**

A The worsening of Mary's drinking does not necessarily make it harder for her to stop, as the extent of a person's use of alcohol depends on the compulsion to drink which is separate from their level of motivation for change. In some cases the realization of the effects of misusing alcohol which will be more evident with high and sustained misuse can add to the motivation for change. However, Mary's use of alcohol is linked to and supported by her lifestyle, which makes change difficult unless she changes her lifestyle.

It is important to note that where a person has used alcohol over a sustained period of time and it is believed they are physically dependent on it, they should not be advised to completely stop, due to the potentially extreme side effects, which can include extreme agitation, tremors (rigors), hallucinations and fits.

In working with Mary's willingness to change, a commonly used intervention is **motivational interviewing (MI)** which helps the person appreciate their own differing views on their problem behaviour. The intention is not to attempt to persuade the person to change but make them more clearly aware of the different options, to appreciate their own doubts and that they may behave in a different way which might lead to change.

In motivational interviewing there are four general principles:

1 *Express empathy*: The interviewer needs to understand the person's experience, because when people perceive that they are listened to, they are more inclined to openly share their experiences. With regards to Mary, while she has been referred due to her drinking, it is important to acknowledge the impact of the events she has recently experienced such as not securing the promotion.
2 *Support self-efficacy*: The interviewer can work to maximize this by identifying the person's successes. Perfectionism often leads to high personal standards, and not crediting successes while paying excessive attention to reversals. The interviewer can redress the balance by emphasizing Mary's achievements, such as that she has a good job and a long-term relationship, which support the view that she can be successful and change is possible.
3 *Roll with resistance*: It is necessary to avoid conflict and the interviewer being the representative of change. Mary may expect to be challenged about her drinking and respond by defending her behaviour, as she does by insisting she does not have a problem, although admitting she drinks heavily. Instead of presenting a contradictory viewpoint, the interviewer might look at the role alcohol performs for Mary and whether this helps.
4 *Develop discrepancy*: Motivation for change is increased when the person perceives a lack of congruity between their current behaviour and future desired goals. Discussing the consequences of continued drinking with Mary and listing the advantages would allow her to consider the role choice plays and the difference between what she might wish for her future and the consequences of her continued current behaviour.

(Miller and Rollnick 2002)

Mary still feels she does not have a problem with alcohol and expresses reluctance to change, saying that to avoid alcohol would involve a complete change, and although she has had a rough patch, she loves her job and cannot be sure that making a change would produce sufficient rewards to justify the effort.

Often unhelpful behaviours are maintained by lifestyle. Bringing about change can entail a significant disruption in the way the person leads their life, which in turn requires significant motivation and confidence in the prospect of success and the attractiveness of the long-term benefits. In contrast to this, just carrying on as we are can seem more attractive, yet in Mary's case this involves risks to her physical and mental health and may place a strain on her relationship with Martin.

An intervention which might help is a drinking diary, an example of which is given in Table 12.4. It can be difficult for people to identify exactly how much alcohol they consume, and often people drink more than they realize. Through seeing this evidence Mary will be

Table 12.4 A drinking diary

Day	Amount and type of alcohol	Time started and time ended	Who was I with?	Where was I?	Number of units	Cost £	Thoughts/ feelings
Monday		Started: Ended:					
Tuesday		Started: Ended:					
Wednesday		Started: Ended:					
Thursday		Started: Ended:					
Friday		Started: Ended:					
Saturday		Started: Ended:					
Sunday		Started: Ended:					

Source: Adapted from Kipping (2005).

empowered to recognize how much she drinks over time. Often this knowledge helps people's motivation to instigate useful lifestyle changes.

In Mary's case, the effects of stress and life events have led to an increase in her alcohol intake. While it is possible that during times when life is on a stable equilibrium, her alcohol intake might decrease, Mary's use of alcohol to respond to difficulties is not a helpful coping mechanism and has the potential to introduce new problems. Often due to its prevalence within society, issues such as alcohol misuse are masked until these problems impact significantly on the person's life. Engaging with Mary and the interventions used have provided her with the opportunity to review her use of alcohol supportively, and importantly without judgement, as often people experience a sense of shame and embarrassment which prevents their accessing the services which might be able to offer help.

Mary and Martin leave the hospital with the advice to contact her GP to discuss any support she might need. She is given a copy of the drinking diary and leaflets advising on the safe use of alcohol and the contact details for independent agencies in her locality that might be able to help, and of local counselling services which she might contact.

REFERENCES

AddictionInfo.org (2010) Stages of Change Model. Available at: http://www.addictioninfo.org/articles/11/1/Stages-of-Change-Model/Page1.html (accessed 29 September 2010).

Alcoholics Anonymous (2010) *Newcomer to AA: About Alcoholism.* Available at: http://www.alcoholics-anonymous.org.uk/newcomers/?PageID=69 (accessed 28 September 2010).

BBC (2010) Seeking perfection: nobody's perfect. Available at: http://www.bbc.co.uk/science/human-body/mind/articles/personalityandindividuality/perfectionism.shtml (accessed 28 September 2010).

DoH (Department of Health) (2007) *Safe, Sensible, Social: The Next Steps in the National Alcohol Strategy.* London: DoH.

DoH (Department of Health) (2009) *Local Routes: Guidance for Developing Alcohol Treatment Pathways.* London: DoH.

Drinkaware (2010a) For the facts: effects of alcohol. Available at: http://www.drinkaware.co.uk/facts/effects-of-alcohol-2?utm_source—sn&utm_medium=cpc&utm_term=how%20alcohol&utm_campaign=Alcohol (accessed 28 September 2010).

Drinkaware (2010b) Alcohol, mental health and wellbeing. Available at: http://www.drinkaware.co.uk/facts/factsheets/alcohol-mental-health-and-wellbeing (accessed 28 September 2010).

Ewing, J.A. (1984) Detecting alcoholism, *JAMA,* 252(14): 1905–7.

Kipping, C. (2005) The person who misuses drugs or alcohol, in N. Norman and I. Ryrie (eds) *The Art and Science of Mental Health Nursing: A Textbook of Principles and Practice.* Maidenhead: McGraw-Hill, pp. 481–518.

Miller, W.R. and Rollnick, S. (2002) *Motivational Interviewing: Preparing People for Change,* 2nd edn. New York: Guilford Press.

NCCMH (National Collaborating Centre for Mental Health) (2011) *Alcohol-Use Disorders: The NICE Guidelines on Diagnosis, Assessment and Management of Harmful Drinking and Alcohol Dependence.* National Clinical Practice Guideline 115. London: The British Psychological Society (BPS) and The Royal College of Psychiatrists (RCP).

Newcastle University (2006) *Screening Tools for Alcohol Related Risk.* Gateshead Council: Design Services. Available at: http://www.ncl.ac.uk/ihs/assets/pdfs/hmitm/screeningtools.pdf (accessed 28 September 2010).

NICE (National Institute for Health and Clinical Excellence) (2010) *Alcohol-Use Disorders: Preventing the Development of Hazardous and Harmful Drinking.* NICE Public Health Guidance 24. London: NICE. Available at: http://www.nice.org.uk/nicemedia/live/13001/48984/48984.pdf (accessed 28 September 2010).

Prochaska, J.O. and DiClemente, C.C. (1986) Toward a comprehensive model of change, in W.R. Miller and N. Heather (eds) *Treating Addictive Behaviours: Processes of Change.* New York: Plenum Press.

Rogers, C. (1983) *Freedom to Learn for the 80s.* Columbus: Merrill.

WHO (World Health Organization) (2001) *Audit: The Alcohol Use Disorders Identification Test: Guidelines for Use in Primary Care.* 2nd edn. Geneva: WHO.

FURTHER READING

Lesco, P. (2010) Alcoholism: Is it learned or hereditary? Available at: http://www.ehow.co.uk/about_6330905_alcoholism_-learned-hereditary_.html (accessed 28 September 2010).

Motivational Interviewing: Resources for Clinicians, Researchers and Trainers. Available at: http://www.motivationalinterview.org/clinical/principles.html (accessed 27 September 2010).

Substance misuse
May Baker

Richie is 19 years old. His parents divorced when he was 10 and he has had little contact with his father since then. Recently he has been living with his mother, stepfather and 4-year-old sister. Over the past two years relations have been very strained in the household and Richie moved out.

After staying with a friend for a few months he decided to move to another city for a fresh break. He is now homeless and living rough but intermittently seeks shelter in one of the homeless hostels. Richie has made loose friendships with some of the other younger residents in the hostel who use significant amounts of illicit drugs, and through these peer relationships Richie has gravitated towards smoking **heroin**. He sleeps 'rough' most nights and on one occasion Richie was approached by a **homeless outreach worker** who tried to offer some support (NTA 2002b).

There are many concerns for Richie from a physical, psychological and social perspective. This case study will endeavour to address these issues and offer guidance and points for reflection to help assess and implement a collaborative plan for Richie.

Drug use, whether illegal or prescribed, can cause serious problems for the user. Drugs are classified in two ways: by *effects* and *legislation*.

EFFECTS

1 **What are the physical and psychological effects of drug misuse?**

A There are several types of drugs which are taken for their effects on the central nervous system (CNS) and these are classified as: **depressants, hallucinogens** and **stimulants**. These substances all affect the CNS in different ways.

- *Depressants* act on the CNS to decrease brain activity and can make the user feel drowsy and calm. They also help to reduce pain (Wilson 2011).
- *Hallucinogens* disrupt the interaction of nerve cells and the neurotransmitter serotonin to distort perception, and can make the user see strange shapes or vivid colours (Fantegrossi et al. 2007).
- *Stimulants* increase brain activity through their effect on the CNS, and can make the user feel more alert and energetic.

It is important to note that the effects of drugs vary from person to person and consideration should be taken with regards to:

- the type of drug;
- how it is taken;
- the environment in which it is taken.

Mixing drugs can also sometimes have catastrophic effects for the user. For instance, if the user takes heroin, alcohol and valium, they are potentially vulnerable to overdose as these are all depressants as they all inhibit the action of the CNS and may cause respiratory arrest and death.

LEGISLATION

Drugs are controlled under the **Misuse of Drugs Act (1971)**. This Act provides legal regulation for and control of drugs that are banned in the UK and grades them in order of severity to the user and to the public.

The three classes of drugs are **Class A, Class B**, and **Class C** (Table 13.1) and they are classified depending on their harmfulness. There is no clear definition as to why one drug may be more harmful than another; however, certain criteria are used, such as its effects, misuse and social problems. More importantly the categorization of the drug also greatly influences the criminal penalty for its use or sale.

Richie is smoking heroin which is from the family of drugs known as opiates. It is obtained from the scored seed heads of the opium poppy and is mainly grown in Afghanistan and

Table 13.1 Drug classification

Legality		
Class A drugs	*Class B drugs*	*Class C drugs*
Opiates (heroin)	Amphetamine (Class A if	Benzodiazepines (unless
Cocaine	prepared for injecting)	prescribed)
Crack cocaine	Cannabis	Ketamine
Ecstasy	Mephedrone	Anabolic steroids
LSD		GHB
Psilocybin (magic mushrooms)		
Effects		
Stimulants	*Depressants*	*Hallucinogens*
Cocaine	Opiates (heroin)	Psilocybin
Crack cocaine	Alcohol (legal drug)	Ketamine
Amphetamine	Solvents (semi-legal)	LSD
Mephedrone	GHB	Cannabis (also depressant)
Ecstasy	Cannabis (also hallucinogenic)	

Source: Pycroft (2010); Wilson (2011).

Table 13.2 The physical signs of heroin withdrawal

Sweating	Nausea and stomach cramps
Yawning	Diarrhoea and vomiting
Runny nose	Muscle aches
Dilated pupils	Crawling sensation under the skin and scratching
Anxiety and irritability	Difficulty sleeping

Pakistan. The drug is usually a reddish-brown colour and can be smoked, snorted or injected. It is normally sold in small packages called 'bags'. These contain approximately £10 worth of the drug and weigh approximately ¼ of a gram. It is difficult to measure exactly how much pure heroin is in this bag as it is adulterated with other substances to increase bulk, therefore making the drug dealer more money (Wilson 2011). It has many street names depending on the region but the most common are smack, gear and brown. Heroin is smoked by placing it on a piece of tinfoil, heating it underneath (usually with a lighter) until smoke is emitted. This is then inhaled through a tube (rolled-up piece of paper), and the effects are almost instantaneous as it is taken into the CNS through the lungs. This is sometimes referred to as 'chasing the dragon'.

Heroin is a Class A drug and is highly addictive and within a period of time, as brief as a few weeks, Richie will become physically dependent and show signs of this by experiencing physical **heroin withdrawal** symptoms when he is unable to get his normal daily dose (Table 13.2). There is potential for serious harm due to the addictiveness of the drug (DoH 2009). For further information on drugs and their effects, see: http://www.talktofrank.com/drugs.aspx?id=186#effects.

Heroin use is still relatively unusual in the population in the UK, as a whole and even less common in young people, and estimated use of heroin in England and Wales is around 0.7 per cent of 16–19-year-olds, and a little lower in Northern Ireland at 0.5 per cent. However, Scotland appears to have a more serious problem with the drug as the rate is double that of the regions at 1.2 per cent (Hoare 2009). Cannabis is the most frequently used illicit drug in the UK. However, for the majority of young people who try drugs, their experience is brief and often a passing phase but some people go on to have problems (NTA 2002a).

Richie can be regarded as a vulnerable young person as he has lost touch with his family, is homeless and using heroin. National policy states that the government are striving to help and assist young people such as Richie and families who are affected by drug misuse (HM Government 2008; Public Health Wales NHS Trust 2010). The policy is set out in a 10-year strategy and looks at ways in which young people can be identified as being at risk through early detection, intervention and support (HM Government 2008). The main aim is to avoid young people developing long-term drug problems.

ENGAGEMENT

2 **How might the homeless outreach worker engage with Richie?**

A In communication with Richie, the outreach worker may have to initiate communication and try to get to know him, not as a homeless drug user but as a young person, who would have had and may still have dreams and aspirations. Therefore, it is important to avoid appearing patronising or overtly sympathetic in engagement. Instead engagement is about empathy and understanding and allowing self-efficacy through mutual respect and support.

Richie has engaged quite openly with the outreach worker; however, for some young people, this can be difficult. They may be reluctant, due to the often illegal nature of substance misuse and associated activity, or find it difficult to speak to someone who wants to help, or they may just see the outreach worker as intrusive. The young person could also feel vulnerable and ashamed of talking about their drug use and lifestyle.

Engagement is a two-way process and therefore the outreach worker could disclose some of their experiences too, although professional boundaries should always be kept. However, it is vital to be natural, compassionate and non-judgemental. Young people are good at picking up cues when someone is not being genuine and it is important to try to be empathic and consider the person's situation. Sometimes exchanging stories or chatting about interests is a good way to get to know someone and to break the ice. Humour can also help in some instances, but this needs to be carefully judged. The least appropriate way to engage would be that of questioning and judging, even if it is for the person's benefit. It is best not to ask lots of questions in the first few meetings as this tends to instil suspicion and fear and is the least likely way to bring them into services (Langham and Davy 2010).

3   **Reflecting on Richie's situation, how can risk factors be minimized?**

A   The risk factors in drug use are shown in Table 13.3. The homeless outreach worker was fairly successful in engaging with Richie and has found out that he had been experimenting with different drugs when he was at home (cigarettes, alcohol and cannabis). This led to arguments with his mum and when his stepfather found out, he was asked to leave the house which Richie feels was an excuse to get rid of him. He has had some phone contact with his mum who is worried about him.

Table 13.3 Risk factors in drug use

Health problems	If injecting drugs	Social and psychological problems
Risk of overdose	Risk of blood-borne diseases such as HIV and hepatitis	Criminal activity
		Sexually transmitted infections/
Addiction and tolerance	Risk of blood clots and circulatory problems	sexual exploitation
		Family breakdown
Poor diet/dental hygiene	Pulmonary embolisms	Unemployment
	Collapsed veins	Lack of further education
	Infections and abscesses	Mental health problems
		Lack of motivation and enthusiasm
		Increased apathy/low self-esteem

ASSESSMENT

Although various drug **assessment** tools can help to identify and determine drug use and dependency, gathering information from a young person may be difficult especially in Richie's case. The worker does not want to strain the newly formed relationship with him but to foster and encourage openness and trust.

Assessment is a process of gathering information to explore the person's experience and to find out about what is their reality. Screening and assessment tools can have many questions which may take a long time to complete. Some of these questions are personal and emotive, therefore identifying which tool to use and which question to ask is vital when trying to determine risk. Having time to fully complete an assessment in the initial meeting would be beneficial; however, the reality may mean that the assessment is completed over several meetings. Therefore, the worker needs to be flexible, supportive and understanding when making the assessment. The worker will have to use their skill in determining the immediate needs/risks for Richie and focus on these initially.

The assessor may need to measure the problem the person is experiencing by using a set of criteria. In Richie's case, a suitable tool for measuring the severity of his drug use and determining the scale of the problem would be the Severity of Dependence Scale (SDS) (Gossop et al. 1992).

When completing a drug assessment, the worker should ensure that a comprehensive drug history is taken. This will include:

- current drugs used;
- main drug used;
- how much is being used?;
- by which route (i.e. smoked, snorted, injected, etc.)?;
- how often (i.e. daily, weekly)?;
- if daily, how many times a day?;
- do you experience withdrawal symptoms, if so, when and how do they feel?;
- how much do you buy/pay for the drug?;
- how do you fund your drug use?;
- when was the last time you had a drug-free day?

(Preston 1996)

The next process is to try and make sense of this information and collaboratively work with Richie to determine a plan of action. The aim of this plan, when implemented, is to alleviate distress or eliminate the problem (Norman and Ryrie 2004; Barker 2009).

Richie and his outreach worker attended an appointment with the community drug clinic, where he had an initial assessment using the SDS tool (Gossop et al. 1992). **Urinalysis** was taken to identify which drugs were present in his system. Opiates were the only substance identified in his body and he maintained that he ingested it by smoking. He was seen by the clinic doctor for a physical and psychological examination. Fortunately Richie has no physical health needs; however, his social situation means that he is vulnerable to exploitation and exposed to others injecting heroin. He was very reluctant to tell the worker and the doctor how he funds his £30 per day habit. Part of the initial plan is to offer him a prescription for the substitute drug, **methadone** (DoH 2009; British Medical Association 2011). Richie agreed to this prescription and feels that it will help him to find a bit of stability and might help him to stop using heroin altogether.

Most drug clinics screen service users for several substances such as opiates, methadone, cocaine, amphetamine and benzodiazepines. The reason for undertaking a urinalysis is twofold. This confirms that the drug is actually present in the body and therefore prevents the inappropriate prescribing of a potentially lethal drug such as methadone. Although the urinalysis can detect drugs, it will not measure quantities, therefore the prescribed methadone is given in a small dose initially and titrated over several weeks until the optimum dose is reached (DoH 2009: 40–50). Regular urinalysis also helps to monitor the drugs that Richie is using and will help to confirm that he is taking his methadone and if he has stopped using heroin. Some drug workers over-emphasize the importance of urinalysis. This is a good tool as it helps to support verbal confirmation of drug use; however, it is not immune to default and can give false positives. Therefore, it is important for the worker to realize that it should be used as an aid to support the service user and not used as a form of punishment.

Providing Richie with a prescription for methadone can help him regain some stability in his life as he will not need to rely on buying street heroin; it will also help to keep him in contact with services. More importantly, pharmacological management should not be used in isolation. Part of this plan would always include psychosocial interventions, risk management and **relapse prevention**, all of which should be implemented within a clear pathway, involving, where necessary, multi-agency working (DoH 2009).

Richie has been seeing the outreach worker for a few weeks and is happy to receive help. However, he is still using the shelter when he can and is still involved with some of the younger residents there, many of whom are still injecting heroin. Therefore there are still concerns for Richie, such as the risk of overdose, especially if he decides to inject heroin, and the involvement with criminal activities, if he needs to fund his drug use. He obtains his daily prescription of methadone at a local pharmacy and says this really helps him as it stops any withdrawal symptoms. However, he still smokes heroin, usually twice or three times a week. He states the reason for this is boredom as there is little else to do either on the streets or in the hostel. The clinic doctor and his worker are also concerned about his mental well-being, as he appears to be feeling quite despondent and hopeless for the future. He says he misses his mum and his life back home. He is frightened in the hostel and wants to stop using heroin before it ruins his life. He tells his worker that he doesn't want to end up like some of the other guys he has met. He just wants to go home but doesn't know how.

AGREEING AND IMPLEMENTING A PLAN

The government document, *Drugs: Protecting Families and Communities* is the newest drug strategy which endeavours to have a more family and community focus. The aim is to have a 'society free of the problems caused by drugs'. Part of this strategy is to ensure that families and communities are given the support to help tackle and prevent drug use. This may be through enforcement, prevention and treatment with the overall aim of increasing awareness, breaking down boundaries and communicating effectively in tackling drug use within communities.

Part of Richie's plan is reconciliation with his family. This approach will help in several ways:

1 Provide the emotional support and stability that he is lacking.
2 Help him to stay off drugs as he will be moving out of his present environment.
3 Help him to look toward a future (education and/or employment).

Of course, there were reasons why he left the family home initially, and these need to be addressed and tackled prior to re-engaging with his mum and stepfather. To achieve Richie's plan the outreach worker needs to work collaboratively with other services.

COLLABORATIVE WORKING: INTEGRATED CARE

Working together with other professionals is part of integrated care which will assist in achieving the best outcome for the service user by utilizing resources, skills and knowledge from multi-disciplinary services and teams. Best practice dictates that Richie should be offered a place in a **residential detoxification centre**. This could give him a safe and secure environment in which to detoxify from heroin and also meet other needs such as accommodation and education. He will have an assessment of his mental health needs and this environment could offer him enough space and time to get to grips with his problem and identify a structured supported plan for his future needs (NICE 2005; DoH 2009).

Richie's outreach worker suggests that he consider an inpatient detox in a selected residential setting. This would give him time to detoxify safely and make contact and re-engage with his family. He is a little concerned about this as he does not want his mum and stepdad to know of his problem as they would not understand and this would lead to further rejection. His worker tries to convince Richie that rather than focus on the negative he should think of them as his support and that if the situation was explained to them, then they would understand and want to help.

The worker has now really got to know Richie quite well and has determined his motivation to change his situation. Prochaska and DiClemente (1986) describe a **model for behaviour change** (Figure 13.1). Richie is actually doing something about his situation and trying to make changes, therefore, he is between stages 3 and 4, the action and making changes stages.

The worker is keen to re-establish Richie's links with his family as she knows that this could increase his chances of recovery. Although families can be the root of the problem for many young people (such as abuse, neglect and over-protection), they can also be the bedrock of stability and can offer structure, protection, love and support (DoH 2009).

1 Pre-contemplation – not recognizing the problem

2 Contemplation – recognition

3 Action – doing something about it

4 Making changes – attempting behaviour change

5 Maintaining change – keeping this going

6 Relapse – returning to the original behaviour

Figure 13.1 Prochaska and DiClemente's (1986) model for behaviour change

Richie is halfway through completing a heroin **detoxification** in a residential clinic. He is completing this detox with the aid of a reducing methadone regime using the Clinical Opioid Withdrawal Scale (COWS) (Wesson and Ling 2003). He has also been learning about the physical effects of heroin on the body and establishing new ways of coping with stress and boredom. He has been given an appointment to see a counsellor after his detox. He wishes to talk about his parents' divorce and how this affected him when they split up. He still doesn't feel part of his family and feels that he is competing for his mother's attention with his sister. He feels anxious at times and is confused about his future.

Richie's needs have been addressed within a holistic framework. It is necessary especially with the young and vulnerable to look at the picture from every perspective. He has been through a journey of anxiety and instability and found himself in a situation in which he thought he would not come through. However, with proactive workers utilizing their skills and knowledge, services can provide an integrated pathway in which the young person is given every opportunity and support to overcome their drug problem and fulfil their potential.

CONCLUSION

The journey of adolescence can be fraught with difficulties, indecision and mistakes. However, most young people manage to move through this stage in their lives into adulthood with minimal damage, but, for some, the damage can cut much deeper and they become entrapped within a setting of drugs and hopelessness. This case study examined the risks and problems associated with drug use in a young person's life and how the consequences can be far-reaching. It may take considerable time, resources and self-belief to change the young person's situation for the better. Making sustainable change takes time, patience and commitment from Richie, but the people around him, including the homeless outreach worker and members of the multi-disciplinary team, will help him to do so.

REFERENCES

Barker, P. (2009) *Psychiatric and Mental Health Nursing: The Craft of Caring.* London: Hodder Arnold.

British Medical Association (2011) *Royal Pharmaceutical Society, British National Formulary*, p. 207. London: BMJ and Pharmaceutical Press. Available at: http://www.bnf.org/bnf/index.htm (accessed 25 October 2011).

DoH (Department of Health) (2009) *Guidance for the Pharmacological Management of Substance Misuse among Young People.* London: National Treatment Agency, pp. 40–50. Available at: http://www.dh.gov.uk/publications.

Fantegrossi, W.E., Murnane, A.C. and Reissig, C.J. (2007) *The Behavioral Pharmacology of Hallucinogens.* Available at: http://www.ncbi.nlm.nih.gov/pmc/articles/PMC2247373/ (accessed 8 October 2011).

Gossop, M., Griffiths, P., Powis, B. and Strang, J. (1992) Severity of dependence and route of administration of heroin, cocaine and amphetamines. *British Journal of Addiction*, 87: 1527–36.

HM Government (2008) *Drugs: Protecting Families and Communities: The 2008 Drug Strategy, Tackling Drugs, Changing Lives.* CDSD9. London: Home Office.

Hoare, J. (2009) *Drug Misuse Declared: Findings from the 2008/2009 British Crime Survey, England and Wales* (Home Office Statistical Bulletin). London: Home Office.

Langham, B. and Davy, N. (2010) Working with drug users, in D. Conrad and A. White (eds) *Promoting Men's Mental Health*. Oxford: Radcliffe Publishing.

NICE (National Institute for Health and Clinical Excellence) (2005) *Depression in Children and Young People: Identification and Management in Primary, Community and Secondary Care*. London: NICE.

Norman, I. and Ryrie, I. (2004) *The Art and Science of Mental Health Nursing: A Textbook of Principles and Practices*. Maidenhead: Open University Press.

NTA (National Treatment Agency) (2002a) *Models of Care for the Treatment of Drug Misusers: Part 2 Full Reference Report*. London: NTA, Chapter 3.

NTA (National Treatment Agency) (2002b) *Models of Care for the Treatment of Drug Misusers: Part 2 Full Reference Report*. London: NTA, Chapter 4.

Preston, A. (1996) *The Methadone Briefing*. Available at: http://www.exchangesupplies.org/drug_information/briefings/the_methadone_briefing/methadone_briefing/contents.html (accessed 8 October 2011).

Prochaska, J.O. and DiClemente, C.C. (1986) Toward a comprehensive model of change, in W.R. Miller and N. Heather (eds) *Treating Addictive Behaviors: Processes of Change*. New York: Plenum Press.

Public Health Wales NHS Trust (2010) *Vulnerable Groups; Interventions and Models for Care for Substance Misuse in Children and Young People*. Available at: www.wales.nhs.uk/newsarchive (accessed 8 October 2011).

Pycroft, A. (2010) *Understanding and Working with Substance Misusers*. London: Sage.

Wesson, D. and Ling, W. (2003) Clinical Opioid Withdrawal Scale (COWS), *Journal of Psychiatric Drugs*, 35(2).

Wilson, I. (2011) Helping people who misuse substances, in S. Pryjmachuk (ed.) *Mental Health Nursing*. London: Sage.

Self-harm
Michael Nash

Louise is a 20-year-old woman who has been admitted to an acute mental health inpatient ward following an episode of self-harming behaviour. This is her first contact with mental health services. Louise presents with lacerations to both arms; some are superficial scratches, others, while of varying severity and depth, are not life-threatening. There are also visible scars on her arms from apparently previous incidents of self-harming behaviour.

Louise has been admitted via the local Accident and Emergency department following an initial **crisis** assessment by the hospital Mental Health Liaison Team. Louise had consumed half a bottle of vodka and also admitted to smoking cannabis prior to the incident. She denies having taken an overdose of any type and this is corroborated by normal blood test results. She was originally accompanied there by her mother who did not remain with her.

Louise does not appear remorseful for what she has done. She says she is depressed and angry with her parents who 'think she is worthless and do not care about me because I haven't gone to uni like my brothers'. She maintains that she doesn't need any help with her problems, claiming they are down to 'my immaturity, as my parents keep telling me' and that 'I'll grow out of it with time'.

1 | **How do you define self-harm?**

A | Self-harm is a complex issue and while there might be a prevailing understanding about what constitutes an act of self-harm and what constitutes a suicide attempt, there are no uniform definitions of each. The National Institute for Health and Clinical Excellence (2004: 16) defines self-harm as 'self-poisoning or self-injury, irrespective of the apparent purpose of the act'.

However, acts of self-harm do not necessarily indicate a suicide attempt. Both may be differentiated depending on factors such as:

- the severity of the self-harm;
- the lethality of the self-harm event;
- the **intent** behind the self-harm;
- the planning or impulsivity.

Factors such as severity, lethality and intent might lead one to rate an event as a suicide attempt, rather than an act of self-harm. For example, a person found hanging in a secluded place, where they are discovered by accident would indicate a suicide attempt due to the severity, lethality and intent (seclusion may indicate the person did not want to be found, that they were found was due to luck).

In Louise's case, we have an episode of self-harm of moderate severity because of the following evidence:

- no severe wounds – but multiple lacerations;
- non-lethal injuries – no major arteries have been damaged;
- no intent to take her own life – she presented to Accident and Emergency with her mother for treatment.

While self-harm is not usually a failed suicide, it should be remembered that repeated self-harm is a risk factor for eventual suicide.

2 **What types of self-harming behaviours are there?**

A There are many ways in which vulnerable people can self-harm. We need to remember that self-harm can generate feelings of shame and guilt and the reactions and attitudes of others towards self-harm can alienate and stigmatize people. This might result in any self-harm being disguised or hidden. Other forms of self-harm include inserting objects into the body, e.g. putting pins under the skin, swallowing foreign objects, burning, slapping or scratching oneself. In Louise's case, self-harm is by self-mutilation.

Louise was accompanied to A&E with her mother who did not stay with her. At face value, Louise's self-harming behaviour appears to be the result of family conflict. However, the motives for self-harm may not be as straightforward as this. This is why we need a good understanding of the individual factors that contribute to each episode and case of self-harm.

3 **Why do people self-harm?**

A People self-harm for a number of reasons which is why an individualized assessment is important. In a review of the functions of deliberate self-injury, Klonsky (2006) highlights seven reasons why individuals engage in self-harm. These include:

1 **affect** regulation – to alleviate acute negative mood;
2 anti-dissociation – to end the experience of depersonalization;
3 anti-suicide – to replace, compromise with, or avoid the impulse to commit suicide;
4 interpersonal boundaries – to assert one's autonomy or a distinction between self and other;
5 interpersonal influence – to seek help from or manipulate others;
6 self-punishment – to derogate or express anger towards oneself;
7 sensation-seeking – to generate exhilaration or excitement.

Problems relating to alcohol use are common among individuals who deliberately self-harm. Furthermore, alcohol abuse increases the risk of both self-harm and suicide (Haw et al. 2005). Chapter 12 discusses the effects of alcohol include the loss of inhibitions, rapid changes in mood with poor or impulsive decision-making and behaviour (Drinkaware 2010). These are important factors in increasing impulsive actions where ability to self-restrain is impaired and risk-taking behaviour increases.

Louise's self-harming behaviour is a combination of family conflict with aspects of Klonsky's functions including affect regulation, interpersonal boundary setting, interpersonal influence and self-punishment. Substance misuse is also a key factor.

You meet with Louise to conduct an individualized assessment and develop a care plan with her. Getting Louise's own perspective of events surrounding her self-harming behaviour is an important step in her recovery. You adopt a client-centred approach with Louise as this is an important factor in establishing a therapeutic relationship. This allows you to show key engagement skills such as empathy, genuineness and positive regard, which will be important in reaching out to Louise. A client-centred approach will also enable you to work in partnership with Louise in setting firm boundaries that promote her safety and autonomy and also encourage her to be responsible for her actions.

4 **What would a care plan for Louise include?**

A Initially the care plan for Louise would relate to her own safety and security. The care plan would also include a risk assessment and a **risk management** plan. The plan would have two goals: (1) to promote Louise's safety and security; and (2) to decrease the frequency and severity of Louise's self-harm behaviour.

1 Goal – to promote Louise's safety and security. Rationale – to ensure Louise remains safe when she is in hospital.
   (a) Develop a therapeutic relationship with Louise.
   (b) Be non-judgemental in approach to Louise.
   (c) Observe for signs and symptoms of any current mental illness, e.g. stress, anxiety or withdrawal symptoms from substance use.
   (d) Treat symptoms of mental illness or withdrawal from substances by administering prescribed medication under Nursing and Midwifery Council guidelines. Where possible, give medications in liquid form to prevent storing or ensure medications are swallowed.
   (e) Document a risk assessment and risk management plan addressing Louise's current level of risk and individual risk factors.
   (f) Regularly review the care plan with Louise and adapt as required. Ensure effective co-ordination and continuity of care by communicating progress at handover time.
2 Goal – to decrease the frequency and severity of Louise's self-harm behaviour. Rationale – to enable Louise to effectively regulate her emotional distress without resorting to self-harm.
   (a) Keep goals realistic and achievable to promote self-confidence and self-esteem at achievements.
   (b) Effectively treat signs and symptoms of mental illness.
   (c) Reduce risk factors for self-harming behaviour, e.g. by referral to substance misuse services for support.
   (d) Increase Louise's tolerance to distress through education to help recognize precipitating factors and how to deal with these.
   (e) Refer Louise for a psychological assessment or to a nurse consultant in self-harm to begin dialectical behaviour therapy or cognitive behavioural therapy.
   (f) Gently broach the subject of family therapy with Louise as family conflict is a factor in her distress.

RISK ASSESSMENT AND MANAGEMENT OF SELF-HARM

Self-harm is a complex behavioural response to emotional distress so risk assessment and management will be a key part of Louise's care plan. Each episode of self-harm should be analysed to establish the underlying reasons for it, as reasons may change in response to different precipitating factors. Maintaining Louise's safety and security will be important goals in the safe planning of her care.

5 **What are risk factors for self-harm?**

A Risk factors for self-harm are highly individual. This is because not all clients will have the same life experiences or face the same problems that lead to self-harm.

Gelder et al. (2000) suggest that self-harm is most common among young, single teenagers/adults, particularly young women between 12–25 years, people from low socio-economic status, divorcees, teenage wives/mothers and people who abuse substances. NICE (2004) states that individuals with a history of repeated self-harm frequently display characteristics such as poor impulse control, poor problem-solving abilities and interpersonal difficulties.

As part of the individualized assessment and care plan, you conduct a risk assessment with Louise regarding her self-harm. While probing her history of self-harm you find that Louise has taken four paracetamol overdoses in the past. These went unreported as she said that following the overdoses she made herself sick. She claims to have felt no undue effects from these. She also admits to regularly picking at her wounds, sometimes opening them so that she bleeds this way. She says that doing this means she does not have to go to hospital for treatment.

Louise's risk assessment identifies the following risk factors that can contribute to her likelihood to self-harm:

Age – 20 years old

Gender – female

Current mental health problem – feels depressed, anxious, worthless, agitated

Current inability to constructively deal with emotions – anger

Past history of self-harm

Multiple self-harming behaviours: cutting, over-dosing and picking wounds

Current alcohol and substance use

Family relationship problems

Unemployment

GENERAL PRINCIPLES OF RISK ASSESSMENT

Risk assessment is a complex process. However, it can be simplified by using core areas to focus our interviewing. For example, Eales (2009) suggests that, when assessing risk, nurses should explore aspects of recency, severity, frequency and pattern.

In Louise's case, current risk of self-harm is high as the event is very recent, the self-harm was of moderate severity and there is a history of frequent harming behaviour (remember Louise also picks at her wounds to injure herself, but not enough to require help at A & E). Louise may still be emotionally distressed and until this psychological crisis is effectively managed, her risk will remain high as she does not currently have the skills to cope with her distress.

PHYSICAL RISKS IN SELF-HARM

While Louise has stated that she never intends to kill herself, she does not fully recognize the physical risks that self-harm behaviour carries. Louise self-harms in a number of ways which can lead to complex physical problems and this needs to be addressed with her in any counselling sessions.

6 **What are the physical risks that Louise's self-harm behaviour might present to her?**

A Self-harm brings about changes in the body related to the amount of harm done, in Louise's case, the skin has been breached so there is a risk of infection, blood loss, tissue damage and damage to tendons, ligaments or nerves. Scarring will also follow. More violent forms of self-injury often lead to permanent disability an/or hospitalization.

In respect to the paracetamol overdoses, there is a risk of liver damage. However, this risk is not only immediate – during the overdose – it is also long term. Paracetamol poisoning is a major cause of acute liver failure requiring liver transplantation; between 1998 and 2002, 111 liver transplants (4 per cent of all liver transplants) were carried out in England and Wales on people who had taken an overdose of paracetamol (NICE 2004).

7 **How can we manage Louise's risk of self-harm?**

A There are two broad aspects to the risk management of self-harm: (1) the operational risk management (ORM); and (2) the therapeutic risk management (TRM). ORM involves the practical procedures that can be employed to reduce the likelihood of self-harm in the in-patient environment. The two most routinely employed methods are: (1) searching personal effects and removing sharp items or medications that can be used to self-harm; and (2) placing the person on a level of observation so that their mental state, mood, behaviour and location can be closely monitored. Here a designated carer would chaperone Louise wherever she went, even to the toilet or observe her having a shower. This method of risk management is closely aligned to the local policies and procedures of the ward or unit, so you are encouraged to familiarize yourself with these.

TRM of self-harm is much more complex as this is where the work of unravelling personal and inter-personal conflict begins, of where self-esteem, self-image and self-worth are increased, where coping skills are enhanced and where the person develops the life skills to be able to cope with natural emotional stress without resorting to self-harm. For self-harm the most constructive TRM will be harm minimization and risk reduction. Harm minimization and risk reduction represent realistic approaches for Louise as they recognize that resolving the core issues around self-harm are long-term goals, probably over many years. Therefore there is recognition that while self-harm may still occur, the harm that is caused is minimized and the risks that provoke self-harm are reduced.

TRM will also involve the treatment of any symptoms of mental illness by medication and the use of 'talking therapies' such as dialectical behavioural therapy (DBT) and cognitive behavioural therapy (CBT). One therapeutic way of trying to prevent self-harm is the use of **no self-harm contracts**.

Louise has now been on the ward for four days and there have been no reported or recorded incidents of self-harm. You meet with her to discuss her therapeutic risk management plan and she discloses that she is feeling less agitated and anxious. She talks of her admission as giving her respite from family pressures. She states she has not taken alcohol or other substances since her admission.

You suggest to Louise that her mental state appears to be improving and that maybe it is time to develop further plans to increase her coping skills. You also want to show her that she can be trusted to be independent and to manage her urges to self-harm more positively. Louise agrees to be placed on general observation. You also mention the possibility of developing a 'no self-harm contract' with her. You reassure her that she will continue to have your support and that this is a natural progression in her care plan and in regaining her independence.

8   **What do you understand by the term 'no self-harm contract'?**

A   No self-harm contracts (NSHCs) are formal agreements drawn up between the nursing team and service user (Figure 14.1). They are designed to prevent self-harming behaviour by prohibiting the obtaining of materials that can be used in self-harm and the immediate reporting of any self-harming behaviour. NSHCs will usually contain an initial statement in which the client agrees not to kill or harm themselves in any way, and a list of activities or tasks in which the client promises to engage when she/he feels suicidal, although there is little empirical evidence supporting their effectiveness (McConnell Lewis 2007).

Little research has been carried out on the efficacy of NSHCs. However, they may contribute to better partnership working between the service user and nursing team via joint agreements. This may empower the service user to take more constructive responsibility for their actions, e.g. seeking out help when distressed instead of self-harming. This in turn may give some space for service users to consider and reduce impulsive behaviour. NSHCs should also be renewable so the duration of the contract should initially be brief in order to recognize current distress and develop a momentum. For example, in Louise's case, having a NSHC for three

---

I (service user name) agree not to attempt suicide or engage in any acts of self-harm from (date) to (date). (Dates will be reviewed regularly.)

I also agree not to obtain items that can be used to self-harm, especially items such as (include items preferred in self-harm).

I also agree to be referred for help with my substance misuse problem as I recognize that this is a risk factor for self-harm (if applicable).

I also agree that when I am in distress that I will actively seek help and support from my key worker or other team member to prevent me self-harming.

I also agree that I will not hide any self-harm but that I will seek help to prevent further injury through infection or effects of overdosing.

Signed: (Service user)   Date:

Witnessed: (Key worker/Primary Nurse)   Date:

Figure 14.1 Example of a no self-harm contract

weeks will be unrealistic as it does not consider her current distress. Therefore, when she self-harms, it could be a blow to her self-esteem and could reinforce her feelings of worthlessness. Initially a daily NSHC may be more realistic and the duration can increase as Louise develops her coping skills.

The process of drawing up a NSHCs contract tends to be service-driven rather than client-centred and may be over-influenced by operational risk management policy and procedure. This is a disadvantage as it can curtail positive risk taking and promote defensive nursing practice, e.g. restricting activities such as going for a walk for fear of self-harm. NSHCs may not effectively consider the nature of impulsive behaviour, which by definition is unpredictable and therefore difficult to contract for. Finally these contracts might be used un-therapeutically by staff, e.g. over-zealous enforcement may see self-harm service users discharged for breaking the contract.

9 **What can we do to help Louise develop her coping skills?**

A Empowering Louise to develop more positive ways of tolerating distress is a means of managing her risk; it will enhance her coping skills and reduce the likelihood of self-harm. An inter-professional approach will be required and this can involve music therapy as it can be used as a means of distracting Louise from thoughts of self-harm. It may even rekindle her interest in music which might be a means of education or study for her in the future. Occupational therapy may also enhance coping and social skills.

We also need to increase Louise's self-esteem and her self-belief that change is possible, for example, praising Louise and reinforcing her positive coping, when she manages distress without self-harming. An important aspect here is staff attitudes as these can often be very negative and untherapeutic towards people who self-harm. NICE (2004) states that people who have self-harmed should be treated with the same care, respect and privacy as any patient. Therefore, a non-judgemental approach towards Louise if self-harm occurs is necessary. We need to recognize the difficulties Louise faces by effectively managing post-incident emotions, e.g. discuss why she did not adhere to the NSHC or determine what the self-harm signifies.

Helping Louise to cope is the domain of not only health professionals and indeed it is important that Louise is involved in the process. However, self-help or peer support is a well-established part of recovery and support for a whole range of health issues – the Alcoholics Anonymous model is a very good example. Such groups can do much to show people that there is hope of recovery. Having the opportunity to talk with others with direct experience of self-harm, and learn how to cope from peers will further enhance Louise's coping skills and show her that she is not alone. The National Self-Harm Network (NSHN) is a UK charity that offers information and support to people who self-harm, their family, carers and also professionals.

A long-term goal would be to encourage Louise to involve her family in her recovery as she recognizes that family stress is a major precipitating factor in her self-harm.

CONCLUSION

Self-harm is a complex challenge for both nurses and clients. However, in exploring the individual reasons for it, it is possible to enhance positive coping skills and empower clients to adopt more constructive ways of managing their emotional distress. Developing therapeutic relationships with vulnerable people may require nurses to reflect on their attitudes to clients who self-harm. This reflection should aim to challenge negative, or stereotypical, attitudes towards vulnerable clients with complex emotional needs.

Risk assessment and management are one way of making care individualized. These are also dynamic processes, as risk level can change. For example, when things are going well for Louise, she does not engage in self-harm. Therefore, at these times her risk level would be low. However, risk level is not static as it will change in response to life events and living stresses. Therefore, one risk assessment and management plan will not be enough. Risk assessment and management will require regular review in order to ensure that Louise is not taking on too much at one time, or too much too soon.

While Louise's risk level may fluctuate between high risk (in 'bad' times) and low risk (in 'good' times), we can say with certainty that her risk of self-harm is currently long term, i.e. that for the foreseeable future Louise will be at risk of self-harm until such time when she can manage her emotional distress without resorting to self-harming behaviour. However, Louise can feel reassured that mental health nurses will be there to support her on her road to recovery.

The case study has examined the definitions of self-harm and suicide, examined different types of self-harm and different reasons why people might resort to self-harm. It has examined the process of risk assessment and management of self-harm and has outlined the nursing management of self-harm. It has also explored the physical risks of self-harm which is something that is largely neglected in mental health nursing literature and research.

REFERENCES

Drinkaware.co.uk (2010) For the facts: effects of alcohol. Available at: http://www.drinkaware.co.uk/ fact/effects-of-alcohol-2?utm_source—sn&utm_medium=cpc&utm_term=how%20alcohol&utm_ campaign=Alcohol (accessed 26 April 2011).

Eales, S. (2009) Risk assessment and management, in P. Callaghan, J. Playle and L. Cooper (eds) *Mental Health Nursing Skills*. Oxford: Oxford University Press.

Gelder, M., Mayou, R. and Geddes, J. (2000) *Psychiatry*, 2nd edn. Oxford: Oxford University Press.

Haw, C., Hawton, K., Casey, D., Bale, E. and Shepherd, A. (2005) Alcohol dependence, excessive drinking and deliberate self-harm: trends and patterns in Oxford, 1989–2002, *Social Psychiatry and Psychiatric Epidemiology*, 40(12): 964–71.

Klonsky, D.E. (2006) The functions of deliberate self-injury: a review of the evidence, *Clinical Psychology Review*, 27: 226–39.

McConnell Lewis, L. (2007) No-harm contracts: a review of what we know, *Suicide and Life-Threatening Behavior*, 37(1): 50–7.

NICE (National Institute for Health and Clinical Excellence) (2004) *Self-Harm: The Short-term Physical Management and Secondary Prevention of Self-Harm in Primary and Secondary Care*. National Clinical Guideline 16. London: Gaskell and British Psychological Society.

CASE STUDY 15
Anorexia nervosa
John Harrison

Emily is 15 years old and has recently been given a diagnosis of anorexia nervosa following attendance at a local Child and Adolescent Mental Health Service (CAMHS) clinic after initial concerns from teaching staff at her school. Emily lives at home with her parents, Tim, aged 50, a dentist, and Clare, 48, a primary school teacher, and her older sister Beth, 18, who has just been accepted to read Medicine at Oxford University.

Both Emily and Beth attend a local girls' grammar school and are described by staff as quiet and hard working. Emily is involved in a range of afterschool groups such as gymnastics and dance. However, lately staff running the groups have begun to notice a change in Emily's behaviour. They describe her as taking the activities far too seriously and no longer seeming to enjoy the events. Her appearance has also changed, as she prefers 'baggier' clothing, saying that she feels cold even when the room is warm. She has become more withdrawn especially during lunchtime when she will often spend time by herself working in the library. When asked about her lunch, she will tell staff and other pupils that she has already eaten.

At home, her parents too have noticed a change in her behaviour. Emily misses meals telling her mother that she has eaten at a friend's house or comes home late from after school groups. Her choice of foods has also changed and she will prefer certain foods to others, saying that she wishes to follow a healthier diet and refusing offers of old favourites such as sweets and crisps.

PE staff at school noted how thin Emily had become during a games lesson and expressed these concerns to the school nurse who then contacted her parents. A consultation was arranged with her family doctor, despite Emily's protests that all was well. A physical examination showed that Emily was far below the ideal weight for her age and height and a CAMHS referral was made resulting in her diagnosis.

1 **What is anorexia nervosa and how common is it?**

A There are a number of definitions as to what anorexia nervosa (AN) is. However, it is generally agreed that the condition involves sustained and deliberate weight loss and an intense fear on the part of the person that they will gain weight through eating (WHO 2007). AN is, alongside bulimia nervosa and compulsive eating (overeating associated with other psychological disturbances), classified as an eating disorder (ED) in which a person has an unhealthy relationship with food and food consumption (RCP 2008). Such disorders are the most common forms of psychological distress among young women (Wonderlich-Tierney and Wal 2010).

It is believed that as many as 1.1 million people are affected by an ED in the UK (Eating Disorders Association 2006). Girls and young women are ten times more likely to suffer from an ED than boys although research has shown that the numbers of boys and young men developing these problems has risen in recent years. In terms of AN, it is predicted that there is one 15-year-old girl in every 150 affected. Although the condition often begins in adolescence, it can occur in childhood and in a few cases in later life (RCP 2008).

2   **How was Emily given a diagnosis of anorexia nervosa?**

A   When Emily was seen by a member of the CAMHS team, she displayed a number of behaviours characteristic of a diagnosis of AN. These are:

- The issue of weight: in order for a diagnosis to be given, Emily's weight needed to be at least 15 per cent below that which is expected for a person of her age and height. This would have been measured against a graph called the Maudsley Body Mass Index Table. By comparing Emily's weight to the index and giving it a score from 1–25, it is possible to see at what stage of the condition she is at. A score of 20–25 would indicate a normal weight range; a score of less than 13.5 would suggest that the person needs to be admitted to hospital for treatment, while a score of less than 12 would mean that the person is suffering from life-threatening AN. Emily scored 16.5 which indicated that she was affected by AN.
- Other physical problems such as **amenorrhoea** (loss of menstrual cycle) and **lanugo** (growth of fine body hair) demonstrated that Emily was unwell (Orr 2007).
- Aspects of Emily's behaviour also indicated that she had developed AN. During her interview with the member of the CAMHS team, Emily stated that she was not unwell but that she was simply too fat and that she needed to lose weight and that it would be traumatic for her if she gained any more weight despite her thin appearance. The fear of weight gain and a preoccupation with weight and shape are common features of AN. Although the individual is very thin and could indeed be emaciated, they will see themselves as fat (distorted self-body image). They will also strive to avoid any weight gain by missing meals and choosing foods that are low in calories, reducing the amount they eat over time as Emily did both at school and home. As weight is lost, the individual will feel a sense of achievement and this will push them further to lose even more weight. Weight loss will never be enough and the person will never achieve a weight loss goal that they feel will make them happy. This is often followed by another goal, increasing the likelihood that severe physical illness and potential fatality will occur as a result of self-starvation (Hall and Ostroff 1999).
- Emily's choice of clothing too is symptomatic of someone suffering from AN. The person will wear baggy clothes in order to hide what they see as their overweight shape and as they lose weight will use layers to prevent people seeing how much weight they have lost, as well as keeping them warm, as sufferers will often complain of feeling cold (Dawson 2001).

3   **Are there other symptoms of anorexia nervosa?**

A   Although this was not the case with Emily and her family, some people suffering from AN will choose to cook food for others. Families of people who suffer from AN will often experience weight gain as the individual will cook food that is often high in calories while they themselves will eat less and less, almost encouraging others to eat vicariously for them. A preoccupation with the calorie contents of foods will take place and serious efforts will be made to burn off calories including exercising for long periods of time. Individuals may also choose to stand rather than sit as this will help burn calories, though in some cases this is due to the fact that sitting becomes uncomfortable as body fat is lost. Other behaviours include using laxatives to help reduce weight or vomiting after meals in order to prevent calories being taken on board; this type of behaviour is known as purging.

The individual's hair and skin will become dry as nutrients are reabsorbed by the body to support the vital organs. They will become increasingly cold and their hands and feet will feel icy to the touch. Eventually, the person may become lethargic and loss of concentration is a common feature of severe AN, with low pulse and blood pressure a cause for concern (Lacey et al. 2007).

4 **What are the causes of anorexia nervosa?**

A As with all mental health problems, there is often no one single cause for a person developing an eating disorder such as AN. However, Emily does display a number of risk factors that could explain her illness. First, gender is an important factor. As indicated, girls are far more likely to develop an eating disorder than boys. This is partly due to the pressure that society places on young women to be thin. Research has shown that in societies where thinness is not seen as a desirable shape, far fewer eating disorders occur (RCP 2008). In our own culture in the UK, to be thin is seen as beautiful. Magazines and television have been seen as having a major impact on how girls and young women see themselves, with self-worth measured in terms of weight loss. Rates of AN have been seen to be higher among fashion models than the rest of the population (Robles 2011).

Emily was initially praised for losing weight, her family telling her that she was getting rid of the 'puppy fat' she had as a child. Initially positive comments from family and friends have been identified as trigger factors that encourage the individual to make further weight loss a goal, thus leading eventually to disordered thinking about body shape with large numbers of adolescent girls controlling their weight in an unhealthy way (MacLaren and Best 2009).

Emily's choice of hobbies too places her at risk of developing some type of ED. Research from a number of countries has shown that rates of AN are often higher among those young people who are involved in sports in which thinness is seen as a desirable commodity (Rosendahl et al. 2009). As both a gymnast and dancer, Emily would often be exposed to role models that have a very small percentage of body fat. Often those involved in such sports as gymnastics will undertake some form of dieting in order to achieve an ideal weight and which can slip into disordered eating behaviours (Herbrich et al. 2011). Many young women will diet as they see this as a normal part of being an adolescent female and in some cases will believe that strict dietary regimen is to be encouraged (Wilson et al. 2009).

At 15, Emily is also in the age group most likely to be affected by AN. The pressures that we face when undergoing puberty such as the development of adult personalities and roles, can be reversed by the development of AN, physical changes will take place to body shape and this can be a cause of distress to some. The individual who has AN will not develop adult sexual characteristics such as pubic hair and breasts, and menstrual periods will cease. This will allow the individual to retreat into the safe known world of childhood where issues such as sexual relationships and taking on adult roles may be delayed.

Emily has been described as a hard-working pupil. Her teachers have noted that she strives to achieve the highest possible marks in her studies and becomes unhappy if she is not in first place in the class. Many people who suffer from AN place very high demands upon themselves academically and will often measure their own self-worth in such a way (Robles 2011). Indeed, many of those who have been diagnosed with AN will accept that they seek perfection in all that they do (Nilsson et al. 2008). That Emily's sister Beth is academically able is also a factor. Many people who develop AN describe a need to obtain reassurance and praise from those around them and feel that they are being compared to others and judged by how successful they are (Wonderlich-Tierney and Wal 2010).

Research has shown that many people with AN will seek the reassurance and praise of their parents due to their low self-esteem (Amianto et al. 2011). Beth's success in her work has caused Emily to feel that she must work harder in order to stop her parents loving her any less. Both parents obtained a university education and this has led in part to Emily believing that she too must do well in order to please them. Family life has been identified as an important issue within AN. Food can be seen as a very powerful and divisive subject in families and a number of people who develop AN describe refusing food as a way of having control over some aspect of their lives (Kerr et al. 2007). Emily would describe feelings of elation when she had missed meals with her family, seeing it as one way in which she could have some say in who she was and that she could be her own person and not someone who lived in Beth's shadow.

5 **What treatment will Emily receive?**

A Given Emily's age and her score on the **Body Mass Index (BMI)** table, it was felt that she would be treated in the community using a range of therapeutic approaches:

- The first process would involve the restoration of her weight to normal levels for her age and height. This involves the use of the **Maudsley Model** of family treatment (Rhodes et al. 2009). In this programme Emily's parents are supported by members of the CAMHS team to help Emily regain weight by introducing a range of foods at the same time as increasing their quantity.
- Over time, Emily would be encouraged to take responsibility for eating safely. The approach makes use of the whole family and Beth too would be asked to encourage Emily to consider more appropriate responses to food. The theory behind such an approach is to make the whole family part of Emily's recovery, thereby dealing with the issues that might have led to Emily developing disordered eating in the first place. The aim initially is to ensure that Emily is gaining weight in the range of 0.5 kg per week. Throughout this process the family are supported by experts from CAMHS who monitor Emily's progress on a regular basis.
- The family will also undergo a number of family therapy sessions in order for them to come to terms with the diagnosis of AN that Emily has been given. The sessions will take place over a 12-month period, the length of time deemed optimum in successful treatment outcomes (Couturier et al. 2010). Emily too will have a series of individual sessions with a therapist based on cognitive behavioural therapy (CBT). The aim of the therapy is to improve issues of self-esteem for Emily as well helping her come to terms with the issues she has around food and her own body shape (Gowers 2008). A total of 20 sessions over five months will take place as Emily is encouraged to return to normal adolescence.

6 **How are guidelines for treatment established, and are other therapeutic approaches available?**

A As with many other conditions, optimal treatment of anorexia has been established following a range of research studies and appraisal of the evidence. The most notable of these are the

NICE (National Institute for Health and Clinical Excellence) guidelines that were developed in 2004, following investigations by the National Collaborating Centre for Mental Health (NCCMH) (2004). These have been designed to provide a framework for treatment, taking into consideration issues such as the age of the person suffering from AN and the level of risk their condition presents. However, the range of treatments available is constantly changing, and more recent research has indicated that other forms of specialist in-patient therapy may prove more beneficial in long-term outcomes (Gowers et al. 2007).

In-patient treatment has often been seen as a last resort for those with AN with the level of treatment often linked to the level of risk. In some severe cases individuals are compulsorily admitted under the **Mental Health Act** (MHA) (1983) in order to ensure treatment takes place (Tan et al. 2010). Often, for younger patients, this means admission to a general paediatric ward or generic tier four CAMHS unit. However, the development of specialized eating disorder in-patient units for young people with ED has brought about a change in current thinking (Gowers et al. 2007).

CONCLUSION

Although Emily has accessed help and is receiving treatment, often progress is gradual and incremental. Even with treatment, those suffering from AN, such as Emily, can often have a poor prognosis. Of those who receive treatment, 43 per cent will make a full recovery; 36 per cent will show some signs of improvement; 20 per cent will develop chronic ED problems lasting many years and, of these, 5 per cent will die as a consequence of AN (Steinhausen 2002). Prompt treatment for AN is now felt to be necessary in order to prevent the long-term damage to both brain function and internal organs, that can lead to a poor prognosis for the individual with a limited likelihood of a full recovery (Treasure and Russell 2011). Essentially, untreated AN can prove to be fatal, hence the importance of prompt and sustained treatment. While many of those who suffer from AN have difficulty engaging with treatment and often find relapses occur, perseverance is essential to ensure a positive outcome for young people like Emily.

REFERENCES

Amianto, F., Abbate-Daga, G., Morando, S., Sobrero, C. and Fassino, S. (2011) Personality development characteristics of women with anorexia nervosa, their healthy siblings and healthy controls: what prevents and what relates to psychopathology? *Psychiatry Research*, 187: 401–8.

Couturier, J., Isserlin, L. and Lock, J. (2010) Family based treatment for adolescents with anorexia nervosa: a dissemination study, *Eating Disorders*, 19: 199–209.

Dawson, D. (2001) *Anorexia and Bulimia: A Parent's Guide to Recognising Eating Disorders and Taking Control*. London: Vermillion.

Eating Disorders Association (2006) *Time to Tell*. Norwich: Eating Disorders Association.

Gowers, S. (2008) Management of eating disorders in children and adolescents, *British Medical Journal*, 93: 331–4.

Gowers, S., Clark, A., Roberts, C., Griffiths, A., Edwards, V., Bryan, C., Smethhurst, N., Byford, S. and Barrett, B. (2007) Clinical effectiveness of treatments for anorexia nervosa in adolescents: randomised controlled trial. *British Journal of Psychiatry*, 191: 427–35.

Hall, L. and Ostroff, M. (1999) *Anorexia Nervosa: A Guide to Recovery*. Carlsbad: Gurze Books.

Herbrich, L., Pfeiffer, E., Lehmkuhl, U. and Schneider, N. (2011) Anorexia athletic in pre-professional ballet dancers, *Journal of Sports Sciences*, 29: 1115–23.

Hutchings, M. and Thornton. C. (2001) *How to Recover from Anorexia and Other Eating Disorders*. Alexandria, VA: Hale and Iremonger Pty Ltd.

Kerr, J., Linder, K. and Blaydon, M. (2007) *Exercise Dependence*. Abingdon: Routledge.

Lacey, J., Hinton, C. and Robinson, K. (2007) *Overcoming Anorexia*. London: Sheldon Press.

MacLaren, V. and Best, L. (2009) Female students' disordered eating and the big five personality facets: *Eating Behaviours*, 106: 192–195.

NCCMH (National Collaborating Centre for Mental Health) (2004) *Core Interventions in the Treatment and Management of Anorexia Nervosa, Bulimia Nervosa and Related Eating Disorders*. London: British Psychological Society and Gaskell.

Nilsson, K., Sundbom, E. and Hagglof, B. (2008) A longitudinal study of perfectionism in adolescent onset anorexia nervosa-restricting type, *European Eating Disorders Review*, 16: 386–94.

Orr, T. (2007) *When the Mirror Lies*. Danbury: Franklin Watts.

RCP (Royal College of Psychiatrists) (2008) *Eating Disorders*. London: RCPsych.

Rhodes, P., Brown, J. and Madden, S. (2009) The Maudsley model of family based treatment for anorexia nervosa: a qualitative evaluation of parent to parent consultation, *Journal of Marital and Family Therapy*, 35: 181–92.

Robles, D. (2011) The thin is in: am I thin enough? Perfectionism and self-esteem in anorexia, *The International Journal of Research and Review*, 6: 65–73.

Rosendahl, J., Bormann, B., Aschenbrenner, K., Aschenbrenner, F. and Strauss, B. (2009) Dieting and disordered eating in German high school athletes and non-athletes, *Scandinavian Journal of Medicine and Science in Sports*, 19: 731–9.

Steinhausen, H. (2002) The outcome of anorexia nervosa in the 20th century, *American Journal of Psychiatry*, 159: 1284–93.

Tan, J., Stewart, A., Fitzpatrick, R. and Hope, T. (2010) Attitudes of patients with anorexia nervosa to compulsory treatment and coercion. *International Journal of Law and Psychiatry*, 33: 13–19.

Treasure, J. and Russell, G. (2011) The case for early intervention in anorexia nervosa: theoretical exploration of maintaining factors, *British Journal of Psychiatry*, 199: 5–7.

Wilson, G., Perrin, N., Rosselli, F., Striegel-Moore, R., DeBar, L. and Kraemer, H. (2009) Beliefs about eating and eating disorders, *Eating Behaviours*, 10: 157–60.

Wonderlich-Tierney, A. and Wal, J. (2010) The effects of social support and coping on the relationship between social anxiety and eating disorders, *Eating Behaviours*, 11: 85–91.

WHO (World Health Organization) (2007) *International Statistical Classification of Diseases and Related Health Problems*, 10th Revision. Geneva: World Health Organization.

WEB RESOURCES

Beat (formerly Eating Disorders Association)
http://www.beat.org.uk

Overcoming Anorexia
http://overcominganorexia.co.uk

Royal College of Psychiatrists
http://rcpsych.ac.uk

CASE STUDY 16
Bulimia nervosa
John Harrison

Wendy is a 25-year-old primary school teacher who has bulimia nervosa (BN). She describes her upbringing as quite normal, with no previous history of mental health problems or eating disorder, although Wendy admits that when growing up, she was influenced by images of other females in the media. This led Wendy to feel that she was overweight in comparison to others, and that in order to be happy, have friends and be popular, she would need to lose weight.

Wendy identifies acquiring BN following a single incident. She describes moving away from home for the first time and being surrounded by people whom she felt were brighter and happier than she was, and as a result she became very critical of her own appearance, feeling that she must do all she could to please others and to look her best at all times. On one occasion after an argument with friends she bought several bars of chocolate and ate them alone in her room in a very short space of time. Following her binge Wendy felt disgusted with her actions, and put her fingers down her throat causing her to vomit. Although afterwards she felt frightened and angry, Wendy soon repeated this cycle of behaviour and over a period of time binge eating followed by self-induced vomiting became a regular feature of her life.

Wendy was generally able to control her behaviour well in the company of others. However, after an event such as an argument or a low mark in an essay, Wendy would buy large quantities of foods with a high fat content, such as crisps and pies that she would normally avoid. When alone, she then ate them very quickly, and induced vomiting after which she felt very low and hopeless. Wendy's life became a constant battle between **binging** and being in control of her eating.

After completing university Wendy was successful in gaining a job as a teacher. However, the problem continued, and often after a bad day at school in response to negative feelings, she bought large amounts of high fat foods which she consumed alone at home, often eating as much as 10,000 calories in a single event once at home and then inducing vomiting. After vomiting, Wendy would feel angry and ashamed of her actions, which on occasion led to her contemplating self-harm as a punishment.

Wendy has recently become engaged to Toby who is also a teacher at the same school. They decided to move in together shortly after which Wendy told Toby of her eating disorder. Due to concern at the effect of her eating disorder on her relationship with Toby, Wendy visited her GP, and was referred to a specialist eating disorder team. She was diagnosed with BN and given a short course of anti-depressant medication, and began a 20-week cognitive behavioural therapy (CBT) course designed to help her come to terms with her disordered eating.

1   **What is bulimia nervosa and how common is it?**

A   BN is classified as an eating disorder (ED). People with BN believe that they have very little control over their lives. A binge then **purge** cycle is created in which the person will attempt to take control of their life and emotions through what they eat (Day 2004). A binge eating episode can see as many as 20,000 calories consumed, after which the person will feel a deep sense of guilt and shame for their actions. After binge eating the person will then carry out a purge of the food which they have consumed, and this can take a variety of forms. Examples include the use of laxatives, diuretics, strict exercise regimes devised with the purpose of using up large amounts of energy, or, as in the case of Wendy, self-induced vomiting (Mehler 2011).

Unlike anorexia nervosa (AN) the person may not be emaciated in appearance, and the problem often remains undiagnosed for many years. Often the person will seem to eat normally in public settings and keep their binge eating and purging secret, even from those close to them (RCP 2008). BN is a relatively common ED affecting as many as 4 in 100 women and girls, although the condition occurs less frequently in males. It is more common in countries such as the United Kingdom, where emphasis is placed on thinness being the ideal female shape (Ruhl et al. 2011). The incidence of BN among younger adolescents has been increasing in number in recent years (Le Grange 2010). It is known that BN occurs together with other mental health issues; for example, people experiencing BN are often diagnosed with depression and personality disorder, and may engage in risk-taking behaviours such as drug taking and shoplifting.

2 · What are the causes of bulimia nervosa?

A · Together with most other mental health problems, there is no specific cause for BN. However, clinical research has identified a number of factors, some of which affect Wendy. Low self-esteem is felt to be one of the main reasons for developing BN (Mond et al. 2004). When Wendy was a student, she compared herself unfavourably with those around her. Rodgers and Chabrol (2009) have identified dissatisfaction with the self, and especially with body shape as one of the central features of BN. Consistent with this, Wendy identified often comparing herself unfavourably to those around her, but also from her youth to images of other women in magazines or on television, feeling that she was overweight, and that in order to be happy and popular and to have friends she would need to lose weight.

Research has shown that people experiencing BN are more likely to be affected by images of others in the media and to see themselves as inferior in body shape (Ruhl et al. 2011). Many authors feel that Western society, with its emphasis on thinness as being attractive, plays a significant role in the development of low self-worth among young women such as Wendy (Le Grange 2010). Day (2004) describes people with BN as feeling lonely and despairing about ever feeling happy, which impacts on their engagement with treatment and positive motivation for change.

It has also been identified that often people engage in BN due to feeling very negative about themselves, and Wendy identifies first beginning to binge and purge after a row with friends (Cockerham et al. 2009). The cycle of Wendy's BN has tended to be triggered by events when she feels bad about herself. Low self-esteem is also evident in the need to seek praise from others, and lack of self-worth and these feelings of inferiority may have been present since Wendy's childhood.

Although not seemingly evident in Wendy's case, poor family relationships are also regarded as a factor predisposing people to BN. Parents who are overly critical toward their children, particularly in regard to weight, may cause the young person to develop confused and negative attitudes toward food, and to see thinness as a way of pleasing those around them (Somerville et al. 2007). Other causes include having a parent who is negative about themselves and has a confusing relationship between food and self-worth (Rodgers and Chabrol 2009).

3 **What happens if bulimia goes untreated?**

A While BN has a far lower mortality rate than anorexia nervosa (AN) (RCP 2008), and acute physical health problems such as osteoporosis are rare, there are a number of serious potential consequences. Alongside the obvious issues of impaired psychosocial functioning, the person with BN can face a number of other physical health problems as a result of repeated and extreme purging and binging (Mehler 2011).

Possibly the best known problem surrounds the impact on oral health of repeated vomiting. The person with BN may find that their teeth begin to suffer from serious **dental erosion**, as the acid from their stomach destroys dental enamel. Gum problems can also be experienced, leading to tooth loss (Ximenes et al. 2010).

If the person uses laxatives, then this could have an impact on their digestive system, as frequent repetition of this form of purging can result in changes to the lining of the gut wall, resulting in some cases in loss of bowel function, requiring corrective surgery (Bryant-Waugh et al. 2006). Gastric problems have also been identified as occurring in people who vomit after an episode of binge eating, while acid can cause permanent damage to the throat as well as the stomach.

Other problems include electrolyte abnormalities, damage to the skin on the fingers when inducing vomiting and swollen leg joints (Mehler 2011). What should be remembered is that the treatment for such conditions is effective, ensuring that patients such as Wendy are able to make a full recovery from their condition.

4 **What treatment will Wendy receive?**

A The treatment of BN has been established by the National Institute for Health and Clinical Excellence (NICE), which has outlined a combined approach to care (Wilson and Shafran 2005). When Wendy was first interviewed by a psychiatrist from the eating disorders team, she was prescribed a Selective Serotonin Reuptake Inhibitor (SSRI) which is the most effective form of medication to use with BN (Somerville et al. 2007). In particular, fluoxetine is considered the first choice drug within the SSRI class for BN. Wendy was prescribed 80 mg a day, which is far higher than the dosage in treating depression (Mitchell et al. 2007).

While SSRIs are more commonly known for use in the treatment of depression, and it is likely that many people with BN will also have features of this mental health problem, their use for people with BN is for a very specific purpose. The intention is that the SSRI will act to reduce the strong feelings of needing to binge, and reduce the person's preoccupation with body shape and weight issues. However, the use of medication is only thought to be of benefit in the short term (Mitchell and Sellers 2005).

To support Wendy towards being able to make sustained long-term change and manage her BN alongside the use of medication, CBT is regarded as the most effective treatment for dealing with disordered eating (Walsh et al. 2004). NICE guidelines recommend that an individual attend between 16 and 20 sessions of CBT (NCCMH 2004). Sessions are generally weekly, and an hour in length and Wendy will work with a therapist to help her better manage her BN.

During CBT sessions, the therapist will help Wendy to come to terms with a number of issues surrounding her BN. First, it is important to bring an end to patterns of binge eating and subsequent **compensatory behaviours** of purging. The therapist will work with Wendy to help her understand the feelings of loss of control that lead to her binges. The therapist will ask Wendy to keep a diary of how she feels before a binge to allow her to identify what led to them taking place, or triggers. Over time, through better understanding the patterns of how her binging occurs, this will result in Wendy being able to practise interventions to disrupt the cycle and reduce the intensity of feeling the need to repeat the cycle of binging and purging (McIntosh et al. 2011).

Other elements of therapy include developing a pattern of regular eating for Wendy. Wherever possible, it is helpful for Toby and Wendy to eat together at meal times to ensure that food does not become an issue of binging and purging, as a central feature of BN is that it occurs in secret and when the person is alone. Furthermore, many people who disclose eating disorders are fearful of rejection, and blame from other family members. Including Toby in therapy will help to address the guilt and shame which Wendy might experience, and help them both come to terms with Wendy's BN (Le Grange 2010). It is also a helpful way of boosting Wendy's self-esteem, by ensuring that she does not feel rejected for admitting having an ED, which is an important feature of sustained recovery (Cockerham et al. 2009). Involving Toby in Wendy's recovery also effectively uses her support network and accesses effective sources of future support and understanding if the problem should recur in the future.

Engaging with CBT will also allow Wendy to explore the issues that led her to be susceptible to an eating disorder, for example, body dissatisfaction and inappropriate comparisons with others (Mitchell et al. 2007). Issues of communication will also be considered, and Wendy will be able to develop ways of dealing with her anxieties to prevent her feeling the need to binge and purge (Wonderlich-Tierney and Wal 2010).

5 **What other treatments are available for bulimia nervosa?**

A While CBT has been identified as the most effective treatment from clinical trials (Mitchell and Selders 2005), a number of alternative treatment options exist. The use of in-patient treatment is felt to be of little benefit for people with BN and a structured day hospital approach has been suggested. This entails attending a planned treatment programme in a group setting, addressing issues such as healthy eating, coping mechanisms and communication skills in order to reduce reliance on binging and purging behaviours (Fittig et al. 2008). Other treatments include interpersonal therapy. In this treatment there is \an emphasis on the individual's relationships with others, as well as exploring issues of grief and loss (RCP 2008).

However, what ought to be remembered is that any therapeutic approach to BN has a high dropout rate, and that many people have difficulty responding to treatment. This, together with the continuing high number of people who are experiencing this problem, indicates that there is a significant need for the further development of effective treatment options (Le Grange 2010).

CONCLUSION

People with BN such as Wendy experience a mental health problem which is occurring with increasing frequency, yet is often the subject of much shame and embarrassment to the individual. While existing treatments provide an evidence-based approach, unfortunately it is often the case that people disengage with treatment. It is necessary to develop a wider range of treatment options to provide choices for people to meet their needs and requirements. When working with people with BN, the support and commitment of the person's pre-existent network of social support offer a valuable opportunity to validate the person's sense of self-esteem, and education of family members concerning the problem ensures that recovery is both supported and sustainable.

REFERENCES

Bryant-Waugh, R., Turner, H., East, P., Gamble, C. and Mehta, R. (2006) Misuse of laxatives among adult outpatients with eating disorders: prevalence and profiles, *International Journal of Eating Disorders*, 39: 404–9.

Cockerham, E., Stopa, L. and Gregg, A. (2009) Implicit self-esteem in bulimia nervosa, *Journal of Behavioural Therapy and Experimental Psychiatry*, 40: 265–73.

Day, M. (2004) The acquisition of bulimia: childhood experience, *Journal of Phenomenological Psychology*, 35: 27–62.

Fittig, E., Jacobi, C., Backmund, H., Gerlingoff, M. and Wittchen, H. (2008) Effectiveness of day hospital treatment for anorexia nervosa and bulimia nervosa, *European Eating Disorders Review*, 16: 341–51.

Le Grange, D. (2010) Family based treatment for adolescents with bulimia nervosa. *The Australian and New Zealand Journal of Family Therapy*, 31: 165–75.

Le Grange, D. and Schmidt, U. (2005) The treatment of adolescents with bulimia nervosa, *Journal of Mental Health*, 14: 587–97.

McIntosh, V., Carter, F., Bulik, C., Frampton, C. and Joyce, P. (2011) Five year outcome of cognitive behavioural therapy and exposure with response prevention for bulimia nervosa, *Psychological Medicine*, 41: 1061–71.

Mehler, P. (2011) Medical complications of bulimia nervosa and their treatments, *International Journal of Eating Disorders*, 44: 95–104.

Mitchell, J., Agras, S. and Wonderlich, S. (2007) Treatment of bulimia nervosa: where are we and where are we going? *International Journal of Eating Disorders*, 40: 95–101.

Mitchell, J. and Selders, A. (2005) Recent treatment research in bulimia nervosa, *Eating Disorders Review*, 16: 1–4.

Mond, J., Hay, P., Rodgers, B., Owen, C. and Beumont, P. (2004) Beliefs of women concerning causes and risk factors for bulimia nervosa. *Australian and New Zealand Journal of Psychiatry*, 38(6): 463–9.

NCCMH (National Collaborating Centre for Mental Health) (2004) *Eating Disorders: Core Interventions in the Treatment and Management of Anorexia Nervosa, Bulimia Nervosa and Related Eating Disorders*. Leicester: British Psychological Society and Gaskell.

RCP (Royal College of Psychiatrists) (2008) *Eating Disorders*. London: Royal College of Psychiatrists.

Rodgers, R. and Chabrol, H. (2009) Parental attitudes, body image disturbance and disordered eating amongst adolescents and young adults: a review, *European Eating Disorders Review*, 17: 137–51.

Ruhl, I., Legenbaur, T. and Hiller, W. (2011) The impact of exposure to images of ideally thin models in TV commercials on eating behaviour: an experimental study with women diagnosed with bulimia nervosa, *Body Image*, 8: 349–96.

Somerville, K., Cooper, M. and Hackmann, A. (2007) Spontaneous imagery in women with bulimia nervosa: an investigation into content characteristics and links to childhood memories, *Journal of Behaviour Therapy and Experimental Psychiatry*, 38: 435–46.

Troop, N., Schmidt, U., Turnbull, S. and Treasure, J. (2000) Self-esteem and responsibility for change in recovery from bulimia nervosa, *European Eating Disorders Review*, 8: 384–93.

Walsh, T., Fairburn, C., Mickley, D., Sysko, R. and Parides, M. (2004) Treatment of bulimia nervosa in a primary care setting, *American Journal of Psychiatry*, 161: 556–61.

Wilson, G. and Shafran, R. (2005) Eating disorders guidelines from NICE, *The Lancet*, 365:79–81.

Wonderlich-Tierney, A. and Wal, J. (2010) The effects of social support and coping on the relationship between social anxiety and eating disorders, *Eating Behaviours*, 11: 85–91.

Ximenes, R., Couto, G. and Sougey, E. (2010) Eating disorders in adolescents and their repercussion in oral health, *International Journal of Eating Disorders*, 43: 59–64.

Young, J., Kloso, J.S. and Weishaar M.E. (2003) *Schema Therapy: A Practitioner's Guide*. New York: Guilford Press.

PART 4
Severe and Enduring Mental Health Problems in Adults

Jenny is a 28-year-old woman who is currently in crisis and who has a diagnosis of **border-line personality disorder**. She has been in contact with mental health services intermittently over the past 10 years but engages when in crisis, and then abruptly disengages with services. Recently, she has been having frequent thoughts of killing herself but is currently refusing treatment. Jenny has been experiencing a range of distressing symptoms, from unstable moods, engaging in self-harming behaviour, constant changes in mood, feelings of emptiness and anger, insomnia, and says: 'At times when I am stressed out, I think people are going to harm me.' Jenny has agreed to a visit at her home by the **Crisis Resolution and Home Treatment (CRHT)** team.

Jenny has three children all by different fathers and who are in temporary care, while none of the fathers has contact with either Jenny or their children. She currently has a boyfriend whom she describes as 'better than the rest put together'. Jenny admits that all of her previous relationships ended due to her infidelity.

Jenny reported a troubled background, and that she had been sexually abused by her father between the ages of 8 to 13. However, Jenny does not like to talk about the abuse, as 'It was a long time ago and what's done is done.'

Recently Jenny has been having recurrent thoughts of killing herself and, when asked about this, states: 'I think of killing myself 15 to 20 times a day; the thoughts last about 30 seconds each time' but then quickly states that she has no plan to do so and would not do it anyway. Jenny's records show that she has attempted to kill herself four times in the past by medication overdoses when she was 14, 18, 20, and 25. When asked what she wanted from the assessment, Jenny jokingly said: 'Maybe somebody can actually figure me out.'

1   **What do you understand by the term 'personality disorder'?**

A   The World Health Organization (WHO 1992) defines **personality disorder** as established maladaptive repetitive patterns of thinking and behaving, which emerge in childhood or adolescence and persist through adult life, diminishing in middle or later life. The *Diagnostic and Statistical Manual* (DSM- IV) (APA 2005) suggests that personality disorder is a group of behaviours or characteristics which cause significant difficulty in the person's ability to function in social relationships or occupational settings, and is the source of much distress to the person experiencing these features.

Personality can be understood as consistencies or patterns in behaving, thinking and feeling, while disorder refers to ways of functioning which persistently cause distress and difficulty to the individual and/or other people. Therefore, a personality disorder consists of patterns of behaving, thinking and feeling, which repeatedly lead to problems for the individual and/or other people. Personality disorder is described as being the 3Ps:

- problematic
- persistent
- pervasive.

While we all have aspects of our personality which resemble those of personality disorder, it only becomes an illness where they are extreme, long-standing, pervasive and dysfunctional.

Borderline personality disorder is a condition characterized by:

- fear of **abandonment**;
- intense and unsuccessful personal relationships;
- unstable self-image and disturbed understanding of own identity;
- impulsive and potentially self-damaging behaviour, for example, promiscuity, eating disorders, substance misuse, or reckless driving and conduct;
- repeated suicidal behaviour, statements of intent or threats, or self-harm;
- unstable moods;
- feelings of emptiness;
- inappropriate anger or problems managing anger, for example, loss of temper, sustained anger, involvement in confrontations with other people;
- passing feelings or episodes of paranoia, **delusions** or **dissociative symptoms**.

(WHO 1992)

The clinical presentation of an individual with borderline personality disorder is one where the individual is often very 'needy' and 'dependent'. This is primarily due to attempts to avoid a sense of feeling abandoned. In saying this, while they present as very 'needy' and don't want to feel abandoned, they also tend to find the experience rather frightening and intimidating. The clinical presentation is also very variable; it is incredibly variable between people; it is incredibly variable within an individual depending on what time of the day you engage with them and what kind of mood they are in. However, most individuals report a chronic **dysphoria** and unhappiness. They can have severe interpersonal dysfunction, tending to have relationships that are stormy and ungratifying. They often fluctuate between totally idealizing someone to totally devaluing someone. One of the hallmarks of the clinical presentation is self-harm; this is distinctly different from suicide attempts although these individuals will make suicide attempts.

The causes of borderline personality disorder may be biological/genetic. The disorder is more common in people who have first-degree relatives who have borderline personality disorder. This does not necessarily support the genetic link, as probably the best way to acquire a borderline personality disorder is to be raised by someone with this condition, pointing to a developmental causation and learned behaviour through poor parenting. It is interesting to note that a large number of these individuals have childhood histories of sexual, emotional and physical abuse and/or neglect. The degree to which this is causative towards borderline personality disorder is unknown at this time.

2   **How do staff attitudes impact on people with borderline personality disorder?**

A   Staff attitudes towards service users with mental illness have been the subject of numerous studies and articles within the literature (Ross and Goldner 2009; Wahl and Aroesty-Cohen 2010). However, literature on staff attitudes toward service users with borderline personality disorder is less common. The attitudes of health workers to people with a borderline personality disorder are consistently found to be less positive than those displayed towards someone with any other mental health problem such as depression or schizophrenia (Markham 2003; Westwood and Baker 2010). Newton-Howes et al. (2008) found that when staff within community mental health teams became aware that a service user had a diagnosis of personality disorder, they believed that he/she would be more difficult to manage. Likewise, results from other studies identified that staff found working with service users with a diagnosis of personality disorder very difficult and many staff underestimate the emotional impact of the clinical work, but also that most staff wanted more training and education on the assessment, treatment and management issues (James and Cowman 2007; Commons Treloar and Lewis 2008; Fortune et al. 2010).

3 **What can we do about negative staff attitudes?**

A These attitudes need to be worked on through staff training and education, raising awareness, and addressing competencies for working with service users with personality disorder. It is important to recognize that this training should involve teams of staff training together and involve service users as trainers. Service user participation in personality disorder training is vital to its success through modelling positive partnerships and challenging unhelpful beliefs. It is also very influential in modelling recovery and hope and in challenging stigma and discrimination.

Personality disorder is an often contested and controversial area of mental health which attracts a particular stigma, even among the mental health services which are there to provide care (Blackburn 2000). Nevertheless, the need for care and services for this group of people is highly evident, and the policy and guidance relating to personality disorders have grown exponentially over the past decade. Comprehensive and integrated services based on multi-agency working have been developed, and there has been the publication of two NICE guidelines in January 2009 relating to borderline personality disorder (BPD) and anti-social personality disorder (NICE 2009a, 2009b).

Personality disorders are common in the UK with an estimated 5–13 per cent of people having problems that would meet the diagnostic criteria (Coid and Yang 2006). In mental health services, 30–40 per cent of out-patients meet the criteria for personality disorder, rising to 40–50 per cent in the in-patient population (Casey 2000). Prevalence shows equal distribution between men and women although the proportions of men and women in some classifications are uneven (NIMHE 2003).

Co-morbidity is common, with personality disordered people often also experiencing depression, anxiety, insomnia, addiction and substance misuse (Swanson et al. 1994). They may also present with eating disorders, brief psychosis and severe and enduring mental health problems including schizophrenia (NIMHE 2003). Despite the prevalence of personality disorders, they are often unrecognized by clinicians, carers and services (DoH 2009), and there is a real need for improved training of practitioners in identifying and assessing personality disorders.

The DSM-IV identifies ten different types of personality disorder and presents them in clusters (Table 17.1). It is worth noting that the diagnosis that is most frequently seen in clinical practice is borderline personality disorder.

Table 17.1 DSM-IV disorders

DSM-IV disorders	Primary presenting features
Cluster A	
Paranoid	Distrust, suspiciousness
Schizoid	Absence of attachment to others, flattened emotions
Schizotypal	Eccentric behaviour, discomfort with close relationships, unusual perceptual experiences
Cluster B	
Antisocial	Disregard for and violation of the rights of others
Histrionic	Attention seeking and excessive emotionality
Narcissistic	Grandiosity, need for admiration, lack of empathy
Borderline	Unstable relationships, self-image, emotions, and impulsivity
Cluster C	
Dependent	Submissive behaviour, excessive need to be taken care of
Avoidant	Oversensitive to negative evaluation, feelings of inadequacy, social inhibition
Obsessive-compulsive	Preoccupation with orderliness, perfection and control

BORDERLINE PERSONALITY DISORDER

4 **Jenny has been diagnosed with borderline personality disorder. From the scenario above, what would indicate this?**

A Jenny would have to meet five out of the nine criteria for this disorder:

- recurrent self-harm/suicide attempts/ideation;
- impulsive self-damaging acts (e.g. substance misuse, binging, and reckless driving);
- intense anger/aggression;
- intense unstable relationships;
- rapid mood changes;
- frantic attempts to avoid loss/being abandoned;
- disturbed identity;
- feel empty inside;
- paranoid/dissociate when under extreme stress.

Jenny has a range of symptoms (mood instability and self-harming behaviour, suicidal thoughts, constant mood changes, feelings of emptiness, feelings of anger, insomnia and 'at times when I am stressed out I think people are going to harm me'). Many of these coincide with features of the diagnostic criteria for borderline personality disorder (NICE 2009a).

5   **In relation to the suicide risk, what issues about Jenny concern you, and how can you deal with this?**

A   Jenny is currently in crisis with suicidal ideation, and states that: 'I think of killing myself 15 to 20 times a day; the thoughts last about 30 seconds each time', but then quickly states that she has no plan to do so and would not do it anyway. However, her records also show that she has attempted to kill herself four times in the past by medication overdoses when she was 14, 18, 20, and 25.

Yet there is a discrepancy between what Jenny is saying and her past behaviour. On the one hand, she has thoughts of killing herself, but states that she has no plans to do so, while, on the other hand, she has a history of four attempted suicides. It is necessary to resolve this discrepancy, and establish Jenny's actual level of suicide risk. This can be approached by using questioning techniques that prompt and probe the nature of suicide-related thinking, and past suicide attempts. But before we explore this, it is important to commence the interview with initial questions that **validate** Jenny's feelings. Because people with borderline personality often have a poor sense of identity and self-image, it is important not to make the assessment an experience which worsens their mental health through feeling judged, but instead works therapeutically through establishing the boundaries of a productive relationship in which Jenny feels respected, safe and able to engage. Carefully phrasing questions to emphasize genuine curiosity and empathy will minimize the potential for misinterpretation while also helping to build a rapport.

Examples of questions include:

* We can see that you are upset, how long have you been feeling like this?
* Do you know why you're feeling like this?

Then we can progress by asking, for example:

* How can we help?
* What's been happening?
* I am concerned about these thoughts you have about killing yourself, I would like to spend some time exploring this.
* Jenny, you say that you think about killing yourself 15 to 20 times a day, can you tell me a little more about these thoughts?
* You attempted to commit suicide before, what was happening in your life then?
* How did you manage to cope with that situation?

From these and similar questions the level of suicide risk that Jenny has can be assessed, while also building a therapeutic relationship.

SUICIDE RISK

Bryan and Rudd (2006) offer a useful framework to use when assessing suicide risk. They reviewed the literature on suicide risk assessment and suggest questions framed around the following concepts to help inform the decision-making process:

- predisposition to suicidal behaviour;
- identifiable precipitant or stressors;
- symptomatic presentation;
- presence of hopelessness;
- the nature of suicidal thinking;
- previous suicidal behaviour;
- impulsivity and self-control;
- protective factors.

Self-rating scales are also useful in measuring the level of suicide intent and ideation and provide a useful reflective tool for the person and the opportunity of building self-awareness and responsibility. Suicide risk assessment tools do exist, but it is important to note that no present suicide risk assessment tool has high levels of validity and reliability (DoH 2007). The role of the clinician is not to be able to predict suicide but to be able to identify when a person's risk has increased, and to then identify appropriate risk management measures (Bryan and Rudd 2006).

CRISIS ASSESSMENT

The initial interview is an opportunity for the team to assess Jenny's level of risk and review current treatment. Although it is important to note that each case is different and might produce other outcomes, the suicidal risk assessment ascertains that Jenny presently has no intentions of committing suicide; and the opportunity to speak to professionals in her home reduces her anger and helps her feel more secure. The team note that Jenny has stopped taking her sodium valproate (which is prescribed as a mood stabilizer) two weeks ago. This seems to have had an impact on her mood. Jenny states that over the last few days her mood is very changeable with her frequently feeling very low, tearful and angry, and she has started to self-harm in the form of superficial scratches to her arms and legs. Jenny states that she feels less angry after self-harming. She stopped taking her sodium valproate after an argument two weeks ago with her current boyfriend.

6 **How can we manage Jenny's crisis?**

A People with borderline personality disorder often experience crises, and like Jenny have a range of symptoms and behaviours. It is important for staff to take each crisis seriously and conduct a thorough assessment and find a balance between intervening to address the crisis and the need for Jenny to be supported to take responsibility.

The aim of crisis management is to get Jenny back to a more stable level of mental functioning as soon as possible. On this occasion after establishing that the suicide risk is low, the crisis team offer Jenny immediate support while continuing to assess her level of risk and review her treatment plan. It was decided to recommence sodium valproate, and for the CRHT team to visit Jenny each day for several days to offer support. Her boyfriend will stay with her to give additional support, and a 24-hour contact number is given in the form of a crisis card and an appointment is also made with her psychiatrist for the next week.

COMPREHENSIVE ASSESSMENT

After the crisis has been resolved, Jenny meets her psychiatrist. She states that she wants to have a thorough assessment this time and is determined to work with the assessment team so that she can get the help she needs. In the past Jenny has never engaged with services long enough to receive a thorough assessment of her needs. This comprehensive assessment can begin once the initial crisis is managed.

7 **How do we provide a comprehensive assessment to help meet Jenny's needs?**

A The most commonly used methods for assessing personality disorder are:

- unstructured clinical interviews;
- semi-structured interviews;
- a psychometric questionnaire.

In Jenny's case, after the crisis situation has been resolved, staff will need to work with her to ensure that she engages with what can be a long assessment process. A large number of assessment tools are available for people with borderline personality disorder, and generally these can be divided into two categories: self-report questionnaires and semi-structured clinical interviews. Self-report questionnaires include:

- the International Personality Disorder Examination Screen;
- the Personality Diagnostic Questionnaire – Revised;
- the Structured Clinical Interview for DSM-IV Axis II Personality Disorders Screen.

The main use of these tools is for screening and not to offer a diagnosis. Several reliable structured interview assessment tools can be used to gather information that can lead to a diagnosis. Among these are the following:

- Structured Clinical Interview for DSM-IV Personality Disorders;
- International Personality Disorder Examination;
- Personality Disorder Schedule;
- Standardized Assessment of Personality;
- Diagnostic Interview for Borderlines.

EARLY EXPERIENCES

Jenny reveals in the interview that she was sexually abused by her father between the ages of 8 and 13. This first began by her father inappropriately touching her then progressed to sexual intercourse two or three times a month from the age of 12. Her father threatened to kill her if she did not keep it secret. Jenny states that her mother knew about the abuse but did nothing to help her and it was never discussed. Jenny recalls an unhappy childhood, with frequent arguments between her parents. If ever Jenny cried, even for a justified reason, she was hit, and there was physical abuse by both parents. Jenny finds it difficult to have any happy memories or feelings towards her parents.

8 **What impact might the sexual abuse by her father have had on Jenny?**

A Early childhood experiences are fundamental to shaping our personalities which are formed from a combination of biological and environmental factors. Each of us inherits a genetic disposition or temperament, which is influenced by our environment, especially in early infant and childhood years. These experiences predominately take place in the family setting and, when positive and nurturing, often lead to mentally healthy individuals. However, when the child grows up in an environment where parents or carers are excessively harsh, inconsistent and/or abusive, either physically, emotionally and/or sexually, this increases the chances of the person developing a perception of self, other people and the world which is negative. These views pervade the person's values, rules, and social and coping skills in what is known as schemas.

9 **How might Jenny's early experiences have influenced her psychological development?**

A Jenny grew up in an emotionally unstable **invalidating environment** without the support neces-sary to foster her normal development, with situations responded to inappropriately or inconsist-ently. For example, Jenny recalls being hit if she cried, and sexually abused by her father while her mother did nothing to help her. Where events are experienced which cause emotional distress to the person yet they receive feedback that these emotions are not correct, or are actively discouraged, this can result in confusion and a general distrust of the person's emotions, with them then becoming unwilling to express anger and distress. As Jenny had no support within the family, it is possible that she learned to be helpless as the safest behaviour in the environment while suppressing her emotion. Often self-harm is a method used to express feelings of intense distress which cannot be otherwise communicated. An emotionally invalidating environment has been suggested as a predisposing factor in the development of borderline personality disorder.

The comprehensive assessment reveals that Jenny has multiple needs. Her diagnosis of borderline personality disorder has been confirmed. The areas of difficulty are: self-harm behaviour, mood instability (frequent low mood), difficulty in controlling her emotions (impul-sivity and anger), interpersonal difficulties and dissociation.

TREATMENT

After the comprehensive assessment, Jenny's level of suicide risk was rated as currently low. It was agreed by Jenny and the team for her to commence **dialectic behavioural therapy (DBT)** which would involve Jenny visiting the Day Centre once a week to work with a trained therapist in DBT both at individual and group levels. This would give Jenny the oppor-tunity to attend sessions on mindfulness, distress tolerance, interpersonal skills and emotional regulation. The CRHT continued to visit on a weekly basis and make occasional phone calls to support Jenny and monitor her mental state. Jenny was also recommended on a mood stabilizer for her mood instability and impulsiveness.

10 **What are the common treatments for borderline personality?**

A NICE (2009) recommends a wide range of psychological therapies of varying intensity, level of complexity and approach, depending on the person's level of need and the suitability of the treatment, while psychotherapy, cognitive behavioural therapy (CBT) and dialectic behav-ioural therapy (DBT) are among the most commonly used. The psychological treatments for borderline personality disorder have not been sufficiently researched to establish which is most effective and more research is needed to advance this area. However, interventions that are carried out over a long period of time have the most positive outcomes.

There is no drug treatment recommended for borderline personality disorder. However, as people experience other mental illnesses as well such as depression, anxiety, and **transient psychosis**, they are often offered medication to relieve these other symptoms.

Assessment and treatment programmes also need to consider outcome domains (how to measure if Jenny is improving or not). However, due to the complexity of borderline personality disorder, no single outcome measure is adequate. Instead it is necessary to use a wide range of outcome measures that include:

- social functioning;
- general well-being;
- cognitive symptoms;
- emotional symptoms;
- behaviours;
- service user experience and harm.

CONCLUSION

Over the next few weeks Jenny's mental health steadily began to improve. At times she was reluctant to engage with the CRHT but has continued with the DBT in spite of finding it challenging and experiencing difficulty facing concerns which she does not like to think about. The long-term prospects for Jenny are that she will continue to experience difficulties at certain times. The priority for the mental health team supporting her is to encourage her to engage for the necessary length of time to enable her to receive help, but also to establish plans to implement in the event of future crises in order to minimize risk and access help at the earliest opportunity.

This case study discusses Jenny, who has a diagnosis of borderline personality disorder and is experiencing crisis. We began with an overview of personality disorder before examining borderline personality disorder and how stigma and labelling are evident even within the mental health services. The crisis assessment focused on the concept of suicide risk and practical interventions to facilitate the interview process and help measure the risk levels. A crisis management plan was then considered and a comprehensive assessment was outlined, together with some of the assessment tools that can be used to offer a diagnosis of borderline personality disorder. Jenny's treatment needs were identified and the treatment programme offered was dialectic behavioural therapy.

REFERENCES

APA (American Psychiatric Association) (2005) *Diagnostic and Statistical Manual of Mental Disorders*, text revision. Washington, DC: APA.

Blackburn, R. (2000) Classification and assessment of personality disorders in mentally disordered offenders: a psychological perspective, *Criminal Behaviour and Mental Health*, 10: S8–S32.

Bryan, C. and Rudd, D. (2006) Advances in the assessment of suicide risk, *Journal of Clinical Psychology*, 62(2): 185–200.

Casey, P. (2000) The epidemiology of personality disorders, in P. Tyrer (ed.) *Personality Disorders: Diagnosis, Management and Course*. London: Wright.

Coid, J. and Yang, M. (2006) Prevalence and correlates of personality disorder in Great Britain, *British Journal of Psychiatry*, 188: 423–31.

Commons Treloar, A.J. and Lewis, A.J. (2008) Professional attitudes toward deliberate self harm in patients with borderline personality disorder, *The Royal Australian and New Zealand College of Psychiatrists*, 42(7): 578–84.

DoH (Department of Health) (2007) *Best Practice in Managing Risk: Principles and Evidence for Best Practice in the Assessment and Management of Risk to Self and Others in Mental Health Services*. Available at: http://www.nimhe.csip.org.uk/risk (accessed 2 August 2011).

DoH (Department of Health) (2009) *Recognising Complexity: Commissioning Guidance for Personality Disorder Services*. London: DoH.

DoH (Department of Health) (2011) *Working with Personality Disorders: A Practitioner's Guide*. London: DoH

Fortune, Z., Rose, D., Crawford, M., Slade, M., Spence, R., Mudd, D., Barrett, B., Coid, J.W., Tyrer, P. and Moran, P. (2010) An evaluation of new services for personality-disordered offenders: staff and service users' perspectives, *International Journal of Social Psychiatry*, 56(2): 186–95.

James, P.D. and Cowman, S. (2007) Psychiatric nurse's knowledge, experience and attitudes towards clients with borderline personality disorder, *Journal of Psychiatric and Mental Health Nursing*, 14: 670–8.

Markham, D. (2003) Attitudes towards patients with a diagnosis of borderline personality disorder: social rejection and dangerousness, *Journal of Mental Health*, 12(6): 595–612.

Newton-Howes, G., Weaver, T. and Tyrer, P. (2008) Attitudes of staff towards patients with personality disorder in community mental health teams, *The Royal Australian and New Zealand College of Psychiatrists*, 42(7): 572–7.

NICE (National Institute for Health and Clinical Excellence) (2009a) *Borderline Personality Disorder: Treatment and Management*. Clinical Guideline 78. London: NICE.

NICE (National Institute for Health and Clinical Excellence) (2009b) *Antisocial Personality Disorder: Treatment, Management and Prevention*. Clinical Guideline 77. London: NICE.

NIMHE (National Institute for Mental Health in England) (2003) *Personality Disorder: No longer a Diagnosis of Exclusion – Policy Implementation Guidance for the Development of Services for People with Personality Disorder*. Available at: http://www.pdprogramme.org.uk/assets/resources/56.pdf (accessed 1 August 2011).

Ross, C.A. and Goldner, E.M. (2009) Stigma, negative attitudes and discrimination towards mental illness within the nursing profession: a review of the literature, *Journal of Psychiatric and Mental Health Nursing*, 16(6): 558–67.

Swanson, M.C., Bland, R.C. and Newman, S.C. (1994) Epidemiology of psychiatric disorders in Edmonton: antisocial personality disorders, *Acta Psychiatrica Scandinavica. Supplementum*, 376: 63–70.

Wahl, O. and Aroesty-Cohen, E. (2010) Attitudes of mental health professionals about mental illness: a review of the recent literature, *Journal of Community Psychology*, 38(1): 48–62.

Westwood, L. and Baker, J. (2010) Attitudes and perceptions of mental health nurses towards borderline personality disorder clients in acute mental health settings: a review of the literature, *Journal of Psychiatric and Mental Health Nursing*, 17(6): 657–62.

WHO (World Health Organization) (1992) *ICD-10 Classification of Mental and Behavioural Disorders: Clinical Descriptions and Diagnostic Guidelines*. London. Churchill Livingstone.

Borderline personality disorder 2
Vanessa Skinner and Nick Wrycraft

Finn is 36 years old and was diagnosed with **borderline personality disorder** 12 years ago. He is single and lives with his parents with whom he has a close and supportive relationship and who both have mental health problems.

Initially, Finn remembers a happy childhood; however, he found the transition from a small village primary school to a large comprehensive overwhelming and struggled with the work. His teachers believed that he was not trying and punished him, while he was bullied by his peers both physically and psychologically, and he made few friendships.

Eventually Finn was diagnosed as having dyslexia at the age of 15, following which his parents educated him at home, and he became increasingly isolated. Finn's family were deeply religious and he experienced acute embarrassment about sexual thoughts and developed an enduring belief that he is bad and has received a death sentence from God.

When he was 16, Finn became an apprentice to a joiner. However, by the time he was 24, he began to experience increasing difficulties with feelings of anger and low mood relating to his experiences at school, and often did not attend work, eventually losing his job. At this time he attended an appointment with a psychiatrist but would accept no help other than medication which he has continued to use feeling that this helps his feelings of depression and low mood.

Over the years Finn has adapted his lifestyle to avoid other people and isolate himself, through fear of their responding negatively to him and confusion over his enduring feelings of anger over his experiences at school. He stays at home as much as possible, engaging in few leisure interests except for walking the dog, maintaining his motorbike and watching television.

However, recently Finn experienced an increase in the intensity of his anger and his mood became more volatile leading him to carry out impetuous and dangerous acts. As a result, he was found in a confused state by the police having ridden his motorbike at high speed through a hedge and agreed to be taken to an adult mental health unit. On arrival, however, Finn expressed a wish to leave, but following assessment by an appropriately qualified doctor and Approved Mental Health Professional (AMHP) was detained under **Section 2 of the Mental Health Act (1983)**.

Although physically unhurt, he appears to be agitated and shocked. This is Finn's first admission to a mental health unit. He is refusing to talk about what has happened and expressing bewilderment that he has been admitted against his will.

1 **What is the Mental Health Act (MHA) (1983)?**

A The Mental Health Act (MHA) (1983) provides legal regulation identifying the circumstances under which people with a mental health problem can have their liberty restricted. The Act is based on several important principles:

- the least intrusive option should be used;
- people should only be compulsorily detained in hospital if no other option is available;
- detention should only be the option of choice if it is in the interests of the person's mental health and safety, and that of others.

There are many Sections of the Mental Health Act (1983) with different purposes and roles. Finn has been detained under Section 2 of the Act, which lasts for up to 28 days, and is for assessment of his mental health.

The role of the nurse is as a carer and not a custodian which is an important distinction and fundamental to the relationship between the nurse and the person receiving care. Often when working with people detained under the Mental Health Act (1983), nurses are in the position of upholding very specific requirements of the law, while at the same time working in a compassionate and therapeutic capacity with people who have been detained and are mentally unwell. This places varied demands on the nurse, and it is important to reflect upon these and carefully consider our interactions with people in these circumstances in order to practise effectively in all aspects of the role.

2   **What are the features of borderline personality disorder?**

A   People with borderline personality disorder experience problems forming and maintaining appropriate and effective relationships with others (Young et al. 2003). The DSM-IV-TR (American Psychiatric Association 2000) also identifies that people with borderline personality disorder have unstable or impaired self-image, which begins in childhood or adolescence. In Finn's case his experiences at school and social isolation presented significant barriers in his ability to form positive relationships. Borderline personality disorder is often evident in a number of areas of the person's life. These include:

- close personal relationships;
- social networks;
- education, occupation and employment;
- housing and finances.

Characteristic of people with borderline personality disorder is the experience of repeated crises and relationship problems. These cover a wide variety of areas and people with borderline personality disorder have a higher predisposition to experiencing other mental health issues such as depression. There is also a high incidence of alcohol and substance misuses and involvement with the criminal justice system. Borderline personality disorder can be triggered by traumatic childhood experiences, leading to the person forming negative views regarding personal image and identity, and sense of values, principles and beliefs.

People with borderline personality disorder often hold extreme, rigid and negative beliefs about themselves, others, and the future. In Finn's case, he believes he has received a death sentence from God. Once a situation has activated these beliefs, even neutral comments by other people are likely to be interpreted negatively, leading to strong emotional reactions, which can in turn precipitate unpredictable behaviour (Beck 1996; NICE 2009).

Finn has been sitting in the reception area to the unit for several hours. He has his head down and has not spoken to anyone even though many people have walked past him. Eventually he approaches the office and quietly asks to speak to Jackie, who has introduced herself as his key worker. Finn says that he still does not believe that he can be kept on the unit, and wants to return home this evening. Finn is very tall and physically imposing and, although in control, appears to be agitated.

3 **What priorities is it necessary for Jackie to consider when engaging with Finn?**

A As a mental health nurse, Jackie's role is to work with Finn to promote his mental health, while risk assessment is also an important consideration (NMC 2008). It is possible to meet both of these goals by creating an environment in which risk is minimized, and Finn is also supported and assisted to engage. Discussing his situation with Finn demonstrates transparency, communication and an awareness of and concern with his needs. If his request were not met, Finn's anxiety and uncertainty might increase, leading to him becoming angry and believing that his concerns are not recognized, which carries the potential of increasing the risk.

However, it is important to remember that risk assessment is both situation-specific and subject to change. Each individual represents a different set of factors, in response to which another approach might be more appropriate.

Among the measures which Jackie might take in meeting with Finn are the following:

- Communicate, discuss and agree the course of action with other team members.
- It might be appropriate for the discussion with Finn to be conducted by two nurses.
- Jackie needs to access a private room where there is comfortable seating and where she can easily be seen and have convenient access to an exit. Some interview rooms have windows where other staff can unobtrusively see the occupants. Many units have purposely built 'quiet rooms' where people can meet with the staff to have discussions.
- Jackie needs to have a personal alarm which has been tested.

4 **What aspects of communication does Jackie need to consider when engaging with Finn?**

A Communication is a complex and multi-faceted process involving a range of functions which we commonly take for granted. However, as healthcare professionals, we need to reflect on the skills we use to communicate in order to engage effectively and therapeutically with Finn.

People with borderline personality disorder often come from dysfunctional environments, and in Finn's case he believes that people routinely form negative preconceptions about him. Therefore it is important to maintain a calm and non-threatening attitude to engender his trust and confidence and adopt a positive perspective and non-judgemental stance (NICE 2005). However, in order to build trust within the relationship, it is necessary to always be truthful, even where this is disappointing or displeasing to the person. In Finn's case, Jackie needs to empathically listen to Finn's concerns and wishes to leave the unit, while at the same time tactfully reinforcing that he has to remain due to being detained under the Mental Health Act (1983).

In considering what skills might be used in engaging with Finn, communication is often regarded as being non-verbal and verbal. Among the issues which we might consider regarding **non-verbal communication** are:

- maintaining eye contact, so that we regularly look at the person, although avoiding staring;
- using appropriate facial expression and gestures, for example, smiling in response to statements which the person finds amusing, or adopting a concerned expression when the person relates an unfortunate event;

- demonstrating appropriate body language, for example, nodding the head in agreement, or using hand gestures to add emphasis to verbal statements, though these should be carefully measured as excessive or overt use may be seen as threatening;
- appropriate body posture to appear relaxed but attentive, and to be situated at a distance in relation to the person that is neither too close or too far away from them;
- the use of comments to signal affirmation that the person is being heard.

Some of the concerns in terms of **verbal communication** are:

- use of a moderate tone of voice;
- asking open questions to encourage Finn to speak and to explain his viewpoint and understanding of the situation to effectively promote empowerment (NICE 2009). Often people feel a therapeutic benefit from being able to explain their situation and be heard;
- using statements which empathize with the person and demonstrate understanding. For example, 'I appreciate that must have been difficult for you', or 'I understand how you might feel in that situation';
- avoiding direct contradiction but instead supporting the person in making sense of their situation;
- avoiding offering or providing solutions to problems;
- identifying Finn's positive coping resources and achievements;
- regularly offering feedback, so that Finn knows he has been understood by summarizing what he has said. This technique also provides structure to the conversation as, if Finn is confused or feeling very agitated, his thoughts may not flow in a logical order;
- summarizing what has been discussed at the end of the conversation.

Effective communication is often regarded as where there is congruence between verbal and non-verbal content. Therefore, while it is necessary to reflect on and develop verbal and non-verbal skills in order for communication to be effective, it is necessary to avoid being artificial.

A further consideration in engaging with Finn is the need to ensure that the boundaries within the relationship are clear. Finn has difficulties forming and maintaining relationships, and has limited experience and skills in interacting with people. While non-verbal and verbal communication will promote engagement, it is helpful to have some clear and explicit guidelines, which allow him to know the nature and purpose of the relationship, and to clarify mutual expectations. Among the range of considerations which might be made are the following:

- Agree a length of time for the meeting.
- Explain the role of the nurse in working with Finn to promote his mental health.
- Clarify what Finn expects from the nurse and the staff. While he may not be able to leave the unit, he may identify other goals or preferred outcomes.

Initially during the discussion with Jackie, Finn was wary and defensive and reluctant to discuss how he felt. He made intermittent eye contact and spoke in brief and fragmented sentences, often not finishing statements. Finn insisted that he wanted to go home, as he had: 'things to do' and did not agree that he needed to remain in hospital.

Jackie did not seek to contradict Finn but discussed the circumstances which led to him arriving on the unit and explained the provisions of Section 2 of the Mental Health Act

(1983), while outlining his right to apply for a tribunal, and describing the role of the nursing staff in supporting Finn and promoting his mental health. Finn became more thoughtful as the discussion progressed. In response to open questions, he talked more expansively about his concerns at the recent increase in feelings of anger and low mood, and that his existing medication seemed to be less effective in helping his mental health. Jackie agreed to discuss this with the doctor, who later saw Finn and changed his medication.

A week passed and Finn settled on the ward although he often spent time alone, and had limited contact with other service users, preferring his own company. However, he developed a good therapeutic relationship with the other nurses, and gradually became more trusting. During one-to-one time he told Jackie that he felt that she was the best nurse on the unit, but he did not like some other members of staff, and felt that they were only interested in coercing him to do what they wanted by attending the groups on the unit. Jackie was surprised to learn this, as she was not aware of there having been any problems.

5 **How might we understand Finn's perception?**

A Borderline personality disorder is often characterized by **splitting**. This is where the person's perspective of their own self and others does not permit that we have attributes which are simultaneously both good and bad. Instead these are situated at opposite extremes in 'all or nothing' thinking and the person often regards themselves and others as being alternately good and then bad within a very brief interval. Such a view lacks coherence and sustainability when applied to everyday life. A view of life based on splitting imposes impossible expectations on human relationships which, due to the range and variety of challenges encountered, cannot possibly endure. Therefore, people with borderline personality disorder often rapidly form relationships, yet these often and repeatedly fail, causing the person and people close to them enormous distress and upheaval. It is not unusual for people with borderline personality disorder to have a history of troubled and unstable relationships.

In Finn's case, he has idealized Jackie and appears to take offence at other members of the team which is consistent with a viewpoint based on splitting. People with borderline personality disorder can cause disruption between teams which leads to tensions, is damaging to their care, and which reinforces their unhelpful belief system.

6 **What actions might Jackie take?**

A Jackie raised the issue at handover for discussion with the other staff and the team manager. Effective communication between team members is an important aspect of in-patient clinical settings in ensuring that consistent care is provided, and to avoid tensions developing. Team discussions also permit the opportunity to develop shared solutions and generate fresh perspectives on care.

The team discussed Finn's care, and it was agreed that the groups were promoted more proactively by some team members than others but, in considering interactions with Finn, these had always been appropriate and amicable. Finn's negative interpretation of the staff seemed to reflect 'all or nothing' thinking. However, it is important not to dismiss people's feelings as being due to their mental health problem. People with borderline personality disorder frequently make unhelpful relationships and Finn has instead chosen to avoid people, and not engage in social contact. While on the ward Finn had limited contact with other service users although he seemed to form good relationships with the staff and the team, set against his background of isolation. This seemed to represent progress, but Finn did not feel this was the case.

The team agreed to encourage Finn to entertain the possibility of simultaneously having opposing thoughts and feelings, and to consider how he categorized good and bad and desirable and undesirable characteristics. The intention of this intervention was to promote greater acceptance and breadth in Finn's self-perception and appraisal of others (Emmelkamp and Kamphuis 2007). In meeting for a routine discussion of Finn's care plan, Jackie revisited the notion of boundaries which she had addressed in her first discussion with Finn. As Finn has limited experience in maintaining and managing relationships, reaffirming boundaries replaces uncertainty and insecurity with clear expectations and defined roles. People with borderline personality disorder need consistency and to feel security in supportive relationships within which their viewpoint will be heard and understood.

CONCLUSION

Finn's mood improved over the next few weeks and he felt the new medication he had been prescribed was helping with his low mood. Finn continued to engage positively with the staff although he still struggled to address his 'all or nothing' thinking, and felt that some team members continued not to like him. However, effective communication between the staff ensured that a team approach was adopted which effectively supported Finn and provided the consistency which people with borderline personality disorder often need.

The role of the mental health nurse involves considering risk and therapeutic engagement; however, these concerns can both be met through applying clinical reasoning and judgement. Identifying and establishing boundaries and expectations are a central part of the function of the mental health nurse in order to define roles and offer continuity of care. People with borderline personality disorder are often regarded negatively; however, effective teamwork and reflection-based practice can effectively engage and provide for their needs.

REFERENCES

American Psychiatric Association (2000) *Diagnostic and Statistical Manual of Mental Disorders*, 4th edn. Washington, DC: APA.

Beck, J.S. (1996) Cognitive therapy of personality disorders, in P. Salkovskis (ed.) *Frontiers of Cognitive Therapy*. New York: Guilford Press, pp. 165–81.

Emmelkamp, P.M. and Kamphuis, J.H. (2007) *Personality Disorders*. Hove: Psychology Press.

NICE (National Institute for Health and Clinical Excellence) (2005) *Violence: The Short-Term Management of Disturbed/Violent Behaviour in In-Patient Psychiatric Settings and Emergency Departments*. NICE Guidelines 35 and 36. Available at: http://www.nice.org.uk/nicemedia/live/10964/29715/29715.pdf (accessed 30 December 2010).

NICE (National Institute for Health and Clinical Excellence) (2009) *Borderline Personality Disorder: Treatment and Management*. NICE Guideline 78. Available at: http://www.nice.org.uk/nicemedia/live/12125/42900/42900.pdf (accessed 30 December 2010).

NMC (Nursing and Midwifery Council) (2008) *The Code: Standards of Conduct, Performance and Ethics for Nurses and Midwives*. Available at: http://www.nmc-uk.org/Nurses-and-midwives/The-code/The-code-in-full/ (accessed 15 July 2011).

FURTHER READING

Being Dyslexic (2011) *What Is Dyslexia?* Available at: http://www.beingdyslexic.co.uk/pages/information/general-information/dyslexia-basics/what-is-dyslexia.php (accessed 30 July 2011).

Benner, P. (1984) *From Novice to Expert: Excellence and Power in Clinical Nursing Practice.* Menlo Park, CA: Addison-Wesley, pp. 13–34.

Bradley, R., Greene, J., Russ, E., Dutra, L. and Westen, D. (2005) A multidimensional meta-analysis of psychotherapy for PTSD, *American Journal of Psychiatry*, 162: 214–27. Available at: EBSCO http://web.ebscohost.com/ehost/detail?vid=1&hid=2&sid=007d722a-9661-4af7-847b-a566d1f70ee0%40sessionmgr3&bdata=JnNpdGU9ZWhvc3QtbGl2ZQ%3d%3d÷=pbh&AN=964252 (accessed 2 February 2009).

Department of Health and Welsh Office (1999) *Mental Health Act 1983 Memorandum on Parts I to VI, VIII and X.* London: The Stationery Office.

Egan, G. (1998) *The Skilled Helper: A Problem-Management Approach to Helping,* 6th edn. Palo Alto, CA: Brooks/Cole Publishing Company.

Gilbert, P. and Procter, S. (2006) Compassionate mind training for people with high shame and self-criticism: overview and pilot study of a group therapy approach. *Clinical Psychology and Psychotherapy.* Re-submission 24 May 2006.

Jones, R. (1999) *Mental Health Act Manual,* 6th edn. London: Sweet and Maxwell.

Kristalyn Salters-Pedneault, D. (2008) *About.com Guide. About.com Borderline Personality Disorder. What is Splitting?* (Updated 19 August 2008.) Available at: http://bpd.about.com/od/faqs/f/splitting.htm (accessed 25 July 2011).

NICE (National Institute for Health and Clinical Excellence) (n.d.) *National Institute for Clinical Excellence SCOPE.* Available at: http://www.nice.org.uk/nicemedia/pdf/BPD_Final_scope.pdf (accessed 30 December 2010).

Resick, P.A. (2001) *Stress and Trauma.* Hove: Psychology Press Ltd.

Taylor, S. (2006) *Clinician's Guide to PTSD: A Cognitive Behavioural Approach.* London: Guilford Press.

Westbrook, D., Kennerley, H. and Kirk, J. (2007) *An Introduction to Cognitive Behaviour Therapy: Skills and Applications.* London: Sage.

Wright, J.H. and Davis, D. (1994) The therapeutic relationship in cognitive-behaviour therapy: patient perceptions and therapist responses. *Cognitive and Behavioural Practice,* 1: 25–45.

Zemler, J. (2011) *PTSD Spirituality.* Available at: http://www.ptsdspirituality.com/2010/02/16/ptsd-spirituality-slippery-slope-of-ptsd-porn-addiction/ (accessed 30 July 2011).

Francis has paranoid schizophrenia. He was born in the Mediterranean where he lived in different locations with his family until he was 8 years old. Francis's family were educationally high achievers, with his father being a writer and his mother an academic specializing in languages. Although Francis's family were very close, they had few other relatives and limited contact with other people and were very protective of their privacy. Francis's mother was a dominant force in the household, had high standards, and was ambitious for her sons and often harshly critical if they failed to succeed. Francis's mother had experienced depression in her early twenties and was suspicious of the mental health services and any form of authority. At her instigation, they moved frequently and travelled widely. The family's isolation was increased as in his early life both Francis and his brother were educated at home.

On moving to live in a large city in Britain, Francis put all of his efforts into his academic work to the exclusion of other interests, and was very successful passing all his qualifications with high marks. At the age of 18, Francis gained a scholarship and travelled to America to study for a degree at a prestigious university and was away from his family for the first time in his life in a country he had not been to before. Unfortunately shortly after arriving there, his father died suddenly and unexpectedly. Francis stopped attending classes and lectures, avoided other people and often stayed awake all night, rarely leaving the room he occupied in a flat shared with some other students. When he was in company, Francis frequently spoke about religion and sometimes seemed to believe that he was the second coming of Jesus and that people intended to kill him. His tutor became concerned about his well-being and persuaded Francis to return to Britain.

On returning to Britain, Francis moved back to his family home. He rarely went out and stayed for much of the time alone in his room. At times Francis could be heard praying and speaking loudly, as though engaged in an argument and often stayed awake all night and slept during the day. Francis's mother was very reluctant to involve the mental health services, and cared for him at home for over a year in spite of his behaviour becoming increasingly unstable and erratic. In attempts to motivate him, Francis's mother arranged job interviews and appointments for him to visit universities and became angry and frustrated when he did not attend them, which led to arguments. Eventually a crisis was reached in which Francis was violent towards his mother and she called the police, leading to Francis being admitted to an in-patient mental health unit where he agreed to remain as an informal admission.

1 **What is schizophrenia?**

A Schizophrenia is a severe form of mental illness in which the person experiences distortions of perception, thought, language and emotions and they are unable to distinguish between their own subjective thoughts and perceptions and events which occur objectively (Glassman 2000). The reason for this is not clear but there is believed to be an element of genetic heredity while environmental factors are also thought to contribute to the likelihood of the person developing schizophrenia (Mueser and McGurk 2004; Kyriakopoulos and Frangou 2007).

Among the features which are often experienced in schizophrenia are:

* delusions – expressing beliefs which are not real;
* **hallucinations** – the person believes that they have experienced something which is not real;
* **disordered thoughts** – statements which are based on delusions or hallucinations;
* abnormal behaviour – where the person acts following their experience of delusions, hallucinations or disordered thoughts.

Schizophrenia is also a heterogeneous disorder, and there are different forms, the range of which is identified in Table 19.1.

2 **What theories might help us understand Francis's schizophrenia?**

A Different theories to help explain schizophrenia include **Erikson's life stage theory** and the **stress vulnerability model**.

Table 19.1 DSM-IV subtypes of schizophrenia

Sub-types	Symptoms
Disorganized schizophrenia	Disorganized speech, constant shift of motion, inexplicable fits of laughter or crying. Disorganized not goal-directed
Catatonic schizophrenia	Catatonic immobility, wild excitement. Repeated gesture, unusual posture maintained for long periods
Paranoid schizophrenia	Persecutory delusions, grandiose delusion, ideas of reference, vivid and auditory hallucinations
Undifferentiated schizophrenia	Meets diagnostic criteria for schizophrenia but not for any of the three main sub-types
Residual schizophrenia	No longer meets the full criteria but still shows some signs of the illness

Source: Adapted from Kring et al. (2010).

ERIKSON'S LIFE STAGE THEORY

Erikson's psychosocial life stage theory is useful in helping our understanding of how people adapt to challenges at all points of life (see Table 19.2). As is the case with Francis, schizophrenia often develops when the person is in late adolescence and early adulthood (Kring et al. 2010). Typically this is a time of great change and upheaval as this is an age when we are entering higher education or beginning working life, developing adult relationships and exposed to enormous pressures and stresses. In Erikson's (1963) life stage theory, there are specific challenges characteristic to each stage. The one which applied to adolescence and which is relevant to Francis is between *identity* and *role confusion* (Erikson 1963), and this centres around the person's developing relationships.

Although having a strong family relationship, Hartup (1989) suggests that in developing an adult identity we need to experience both *vertical* and *horizontal* relationships.

- **Vertical relationships** are the child's attachments to individuals with greater knowledge and social power, such as parents.

Table 19.2 Erikson's life stage theory

Stage	Challenge	Significant events	Positive outcome
Infancy up to 18 months	Trust versus mistrust	Feeding	A sense of trust when the caregiver is reliable and affectionate
Early childhood (2–3 years)	Autonomy versus shame and doubt	Toilet training	Developing a sense of control over physical skills and a sense of independence. Success leads to a sense of autonomy
Preschool (3–5 years)	Initiative versus guilt	Exploration	Asserting an influence over the environment leading to a sense of purpose
School age (6–11 years)	Industry versus inferiority	School	Coping with social and academic demands leading to a sense of competence
Adolescence (12–18 years)	Identity versus role confusion	Social relationships	Developing a sense of self, personal identity and integrity
Young adulthood (19–40 years)	Intimacy versus isolation	Relationships	Forming trusting intimate and loving relationships with others
Middle adulthood (40–65 years)	Generativity versus stagnation	Work and parenthood	Caring for and nurturing children and making a change to benefit other people
Maturity (65 to death)	Ego integrity versus despair	Reflection on life	Reviewing life with a sense of fulfilment and wisdom

Source: Adapted from: About.com.Psychology (2011), 'Erikson's Psychosocial Stages Summary Chart.' Available at: http://psychology.about.com/library/bl_psychosocial_summary.htm (accessed 5 October 2011).

- **Horizontal relationships** are formed when children establish close relationships with individuals who have the same amount of social power as themselves, for example, peers.

While Francis had good vertical relationships, he lacked horizontal relationships, which might have provided him with valuable support following the death of his father. The family's close bonds acted to limit Francis's capacity to form relationships outside the family unit, which are necessary in order to develop an adult identity (Erikson 1963). Even when Francis was an older adolescent and perhaps able to independently initiate relationships, **social learning theory** suggests that the reluctance towards establishing and maintaining social relationships which he learned from his parents was ingrained and hard to change (Bandura and Walters 1963).

Through not succeeding in overcoming the challenge at this life stage, the resulting consequence of 'role confusion' leads to a weak sense of self, and compromised identity (Erikson 1963). This is consistent with what is often experienced in schizophrenia, where the person has difficulty identifying the boundaries between their own self and objective phenomena. However, it should not be assumed that all people who do not successfully negotiate this life stage will become severely mentally ill, as all cases are different.

THE STRESS VULNERABILITY MODEL

The stress vulnerability model of Zubin and Spring (1977) has had an enduring influence in helping us understand the experience of people with psychosis and schizophrenia. Zubin and Spring suggest that an individual may have a genetic predisposition to experience a mental health problem. However, in order for this to become manifest, a trigger is needed. Examples include physical causes, for example, illness, infection, drugs or alcohol. Alternatively there may be traumatic life events, such as stressful living conditions, poverty, family conflict, and, in Francis's case, unexpected bereavement.

In Zubin and Spring's (1977) model, the central factor determining whether the person becomes unwell is their experience of and response to stress. Applied to the case of Francis, he was experiencing several stressors at the time that he became unwell. These include:

- the bereavement of his father;
- Francis was away from the rest of his family and main source of support for the first time in his life in a country with which he was not familiar. While he had moved often, the lack of stability this can cause might have increased his vulnerability;
- Francis was about to begin a degree course.

All of these are comparable to factors in Holmes and Rahe's (1967) **Social Readjustment Rating Scale (SRRS)**, which is a list of events and experiences rated as being stressful. The experience of stressors can disrupt the person's functioning, leading to their being exposed to further sources of stress. For example, Francis's sleep pattern became disrupted which is another factor on the SRRS (Holmes and Rahe 1967).

The family's mobile way of life meant that they did not establish continuity of either home environment or social relationships outside the family which represent significant destabilizing factors. For many people the familiarity of home and the support of friends and social contacts reinforce identity and perform a useful buffer against difficulties during times of **stress**.

EXPRESSED EMOTION

Francis's relationship with his mother while being supportive also involved conflict. High levels of **expressed emotion** by relatives has been identified as contributing to relapse, yet also to the person becoming unwell initially. Expressed emotion is present in three attitudes displayed by family members of a person with a mental health problem. These are: hostile, critical and over-involved:

- *Hostility* is present in the form of blaming the person for their mental illness and being held accountable for negative incidents within the family.
- *Critical comments* are made, which are negative and hostile and excessively emotional.
- *Emotional over-involvement* is present where the relative or family member identifies to a significant extent with the person who is ill and assumes responsibility for the person.

In the case of Francis, his mother has at times been critical of her son, but when he became unwell through arguing with him and arranging interviews and visits to universities, she then demonstrated emotional over-involvement. Family members of a person with a severe and enduring mental health problem often feel helpless and experience strong emotions regarding the person. The role of caring for a person with an acute mental health problem is psychologically and physically demanding and mental health problems are common among carers who may also need support (Sainsbury Centre for Mental Health 1998). Even though Francis has been admitted to an in-patient unit, it is important for mental health professionals to consider his mother's needs. The Care Programme Approach (CPA) requires that care plans are devised for significant others and their needs reviewed annually (Rethink 2006).

While in hospital, Francis was often quiet, polite and subdued in mood. He was reserved among other people and did not form friendships with the other people on the ward, only talking to the staff. Francis was prescribed and took anti-psychotic medication and engaged with therapeutic groups, but felt that the most positive development was his interest in Christianity. He attended a local church regularly for services and theological discussions. Mohr and Huguelet (2004) argue that religion performs a positive function by providing identity and a view of life, together with the social support which can be gained from engaging in religious observance with other people who share the same beliefs.

However, Francis invested a significant amount of time and energy in reading the Bible, and often expressed the belief that he was the second incarnation of Jesus. As a result, members of the local church at which he worshipped were offended and excluded him. As a result of this rejection, Francis was very disappointed but joined another church.

In a review meeting Francis's psychiatrist felt that his interest was caused by his mental illness as he had not previously been religious. The psychiatrist felt that the nursing staff should tactfully discourage Francis's involvement with religion.

3 **Should the nurses discourage Francis's involvement with religion?**

A Religion performs an important and valued role in the lives of many people. However, people experiencing acute mental illness and schizophrenia often have an excessive interest or interpretation of religious or other types of belief. It does appear that Francis has some delusional ideas regarding religion; however, he has also said that this interest has been the most positive development in his time on the in-patient unit and discouragement might undermine the therapeutic relationship. Personal beliefs and values need to be respected, and even if Francis did not have religious beliefs before becoming unwell, it is always possible when a person has experienced mental illness that they can change or gain new beliefs. Instead by encouraging Francis to talk about his interest in religion and what this means to him, the nurses will be better able to assess how this affects his mental health, while allowing Francis to feel supported.

In modern mental health nursing the concept of recovery is especially important. Recovery incorporates a number of principles, some of which are listed below and have relevance to Francis's case:

- Everyone's journey to recovery is different and individual.
- Recovery does not end but is a continuous process.
- Progress might not always be in a forward direction and instead sometimes relapse may occur, yet this should not necessarily be regarded as failure.
- Recovery does not depend upon professional intervention but may occur through other means or actions.
- Recovery cannot be measured by any one theory regarding the causes of mental health problems but instead depends on the person's own estimation.
- Recovery is not a cure but instead can lead to personal growth, self-understanding and development.
- Recovery is about the individual feeling able to take control of their life.

CONCLUSION

Following a long stay on the mental health unit, Francis moved on to living in supported accommodation, as it was agreed between him and his mother that this would be helpful in his gaining independence. Francis is still interested in religion and regularly attends a new church. He has few friends outside of the church but has regular contact with a community mental health nurse who checks with him that he continues to take his anti-psychotic medication, provides psychological support and ensures that he has regular physical health checks at his GP's surgery, something which is often overlooked among people with severe and enduring mental health problems. Living with a severe and enduring mental health problem involves continuous recovery, and increasingly the role of mental health services are focusing on interventions which actively empower service users in their recovery, with independent organizations such as the Hearing Voices network providing valuable support.

REFERENCES

Bandura, A. and Walters, R.H. (1963) *Social Learning and Personality Development.* New York: Rinehart and Winston.
Erikson, E.H. (1963) *Childhood and Society*, 2nd edn. New York: W. W. Norton.
Hartup, W.W. (1989) Social relationships and their developmental significance, *American Psychologist*, 44(2): 120–6.

Glassman, W.E. (2000) *Approaches to Psychology*, 3rd edn. Philadelphia, PA: Open University Press.

Hemphill-Pearson, B.J. (2007) *Assessments in Occupational Therapy Mental Health: An Integrative Approach*. New Jersey: SLACK Incorporated.

Holmes, T.H. and Rahe, R.H. (1967) The Social Readjustment Rating Scale, *Journal of Psychosomatic Research*, 11(2): 213–18.

Kring, A.M. et al. (2010) *Abnormal Psychology*, 11th edn. Hoboken, NJ: John Wiley & Sons, Inc.

Kyriakopoulos, M. and Frangou, S. (2007) Pathophysiology of early onset schizophrenia, *International Review of Psychiatry*, 19(4): 315–24.

Mohr, S. and Huguelet, P. (2004) Spirituality and religious practices among people suffering from schizophrenia in ambulatory care in Geneva, paper presented at 12th Congress of Association of European Psychiatry, Geneva.

Mueser, K.T. and McGurk, S.R. (2004) Schizophrenia, *The Lancet*, 363: 2063–72.

Rethink (2006) *Reach Out to Help Someone Cope with Severe Mental Illness*. London: Rethink.

Sainsbury Centre for Mental Health (1998) *Keys to Engagement*. London: Sainsbury Centre for Mental Health.

Zubin, J. and Spring, B. (1977) Vulnerability: a new view to schizophrenia, *Journal of Abnormal Psychology*, 86: 103–26.

FURTHER READING

Andresen, R., Oades, L.G. and Caputi, P. (2011) *Psychological Recovery: Beyond Mental Illness*. Chichester: Wiley-Blackwell.

Arnold, E. and Boggs, K. (1999) *Interpersonal Relationships: Professional Communication Skills for Nurses*, 3rd edn. Philadelphia, PA: W.B. Saunders.

Barker, P. (ed.) (2003) *Psychiatric and Mental Health Nursing: The Craft of Caring*. London: Arnold.

Barker, P. (ed.) (2009) *Psychiatric and Mental Health Nursing: The Craft of Caring*, 2nd edn. London: Oxford University Press.

Barker, P. (2008) The tidal commitments: extending the value base of mental health recovery, *Journal of Psychiatric and Mental Health Nursing*, 15(2): 93–100.

Barker, P. and Buchanan-Barker., P. (eds) (2005) *The Tidal Model: A Guide for Mental Health Professionals*. Hove: Psychology Press.

Barker, R.L. (ed.) (1999) *The Social Work Dictionary*, 4th edn. Washington, DC: NASW Press.

Bowlby, J. (1982) *Attachment and Loss*, vol. 1. *Attachment*, 2nd edn. New York: Basic Books.

Brennan, G. (2006) Stress vulnerability model of serious mental illness, in C. Gamble and G. Brenan (eds) *Working with Serious Mental Illness: A Manual for Clinical Practice*. Philadelphia, PA: Elsevier Limited, Chapter 4.

Cramer, P. (2006) The development of defence mechanisms, *Journal of Personality*, 55(4): 596–614.

Davidson, L. and Roe, D. (2007) Recovery from versus recovery in serious mental illness: one strategy for lessening confusion plaguing recovery, *Journal of Mental Health*, 16: 459–70.

Davies, P. (2008) *The NHS Handbook 2008/2009*, 10th edn. London: The NHS Confederation.

Erikson, E.H. (1982) Identity and the life cycle, *Psychological Issues*, 1(1): 24–8.

Freud, S. (1926) *Inhibitions, Symptoms and Anxiety*, trans. J. Strachey. New York: Norton.

Gamble, C. and Brennan, G. (2006a) Building relationships: lessons to be learnt, in C. Gamble and G. Brenan (eds) *Working with Serious Mental Illness: A Manual for Clinical Practice*. Philadelphia, PA: Elsevier Limited, Chapter 6.

Gamble, C. and Brennan, G. (2006b) *Working with Serious Mental Illness*. Philadelphia, PA: Elsevier.

Heron, J. (2001) *Helping the Client: A Creative Practical Guide*, 5th edn. London: Sage.

Hoff, L.A. (1995) *People in Crisis: Understanding and Helping*, 4th edn. Redwood City, CA: Addison-Wesley.

Hoff, L.A. et al. (2009) *People in Crisis: Clinical and Diversity Perspectives*, 6th edn. New York: Routledge.

Isaacs, W., Thomas, J. and Goldiamond, I. (1960) Application of Operant Conditioning to reinstate verbal behaviour in psychotics, *Journal of Speech and Hearing Disorders*, 25: 8–12.

Kingsford, D. and Finn, M. (2006) *Tackling Mental Health Crisis*. London: Routledge.

Kirov, G., Kemp, R., Kirov, K., and David, A.S. (1998) Religious faith after psychotic illness, *Psychopathology*, 31: 243–5.

Kring, A.M. et al. (2010) *Abnormal Psychology*, 11th edn. New Jersey: John Wiley and Sons.

Kring, A.M. and Neale, J.M. (1996) Do schizophrenics show a disjunctive relationship among expressive, experiential and physiological components of emotion? *Journal of Abnormal Psychology*, 105: 249–57.

MacCallum, E.J. (2002) Othering and psychiatric nursing, *Journal of Psychiatric and Mental Health Nursing*, 9: 87–94.

Morgan, S. (2000) *Clinical Tool and Practitioner Manual*. London: Sainsbury Centre for Mental Health.

Nursing Midwifery Code of Conduct (2008) *The Code: Standards of Conduct, Performance and Ethics for Nurses and Midwives*. London: DoH.

Orem, D.E. (1971) *Nursing: Concepts of Practice*. Highstown, NJ: McGraw-Hill.

Perkins, R. and Sayce, L. (2006) Social inclusion, in C. Gamble and G. Brenan (eds) *Working with Serious Mental Illness: A Manual for Clinical Practice*. Philadelphia, PA: Elsevier Limited, Chapter 4.

Repper, J. et al. (2007) *Family Carers on the Margin: Experiences of Assessment in Mental Health: Report to the National Coordinating Centre for NHS Service Delivery and Organisation (NCCSDO)*. London: London School of Hygiene and Tropical Medicine.

Roberts, L.W. et al. (2002) Ethics in psychiatric practice: essential ethics skills, informed consent, the therapeutic relationship and confidentiality, *Journal of Psychiatric Practice*, 8: 290–305.

Rogers, C.R. (1951) *Client-Centred Therapy*. Boston: Houghton-Mifflin.

Scheller-Gilkey, M. (2003) Early life stress and PTSD symptoms in patients with co-morbid schizophrenia and substance abuse, *Schizophrenia Research*, 6(2): 167–74.

Spinelli, E. (2005) *Practising Existential Psychotherapy: The Relational World*. London: Sage.

Thibaut, J.W. and Walker, L. (1975) Early research in procedural justice, in E.A. Lind and T.R. Tyler (eds) (1988) *The Social Psychology of Procedural Justice*. New York: Springer.

Thompson, N. (2011) *Crisis Intervention*. Dorset: Russell House Publishing Limited.

Watkins, P. (2009) *Mental Health Practice: A Guide to Compassionate Care*, 2nd edn. Philadelphia, PA: Elsevier Limited.

Weinberger, D.R. (1997) Biological basis of schizophrenia: new direction, *Journal of Clinical Psychiatry*, 58(10): 22–7.

Winterer, G. and Weinberger, D.R. (2004) Trends in neuroscience, *Journal of Clinical Psychiatry*, 27: 683–90.

The carer's perspective

Sally Goldspink and Cliff Riordan

Dave is 18 years old and has been detained on an adult acute mental health ward under Section 3 of the Mental Health Act (1983) due to prolonged low mood, anxiety and paranoid ideas. Dave has no other siblings and usually lives at home with his mum and dad.

Dave was first referred by his GP to the mental health services when he was 17 but over the past year his mental health has deteriorated, causing his present admission. Dave's parents are both teachers and he was planning to start a university course later this year. His parents are anxious for him to recover quickly and resume his studies at school.

During a handover on the ward, the issue was raised about the number and duration of telephone calls to the staff from Dave's mother. Several of the staff expressed the view that the telephone calls should be limited in number and kept brief, in order to protect Dave's confidentiality. It was also suggested that his parents' anxieties are not helpful to his recovery.

As Dave's primary nurse, the team leader has asked you to meet Dave's parents and discuss these concerns.

1 **What issues regarding working with carers do you need to consider before contacting Dave's parents?**

A Working with **carers** requires the same skills and professionalism as when working with service users, and can be complex and emotionally challenging. The term 'family' has a broad range of applications encompassing relationships such as mums, dads, wives, husbands, brothers, sisters and in the extended sense friends and our wider social network. These relationships involve a complex and personal range of definitions and understandings. While the role of a carer is often performed by people who also share these close emotional attachments, the term 'carer' also includes those who are paid to care (DoH 2010). Therefore, when working with families and carers, we need to consider them as individuals, and in terms of their significance to the service user.

It is also important we recognize that tension can arise between our professional perspective becoming entangled with our own subjective experiences, attitudes and personal understanding because we all have people we love and care about, and whom we would find it difficult to see in distress, and this may stretch our limits of coping (Zubin and Spring 1977). Therefore, it is important that we view carers as individuals, with their own interpretations of and response to events, in order for us to understand how we can best work with them and for the benefit of the service user (Glynn 2006).

Consciously developing an empathic awareness of the carer's perspective helps us work more effectively and understand that in every situation, each person will have their own perspective, point of view and way of coping. Sometimes these coping strategies are helpful, sometimes they are not, but the actions of carers represent their best attempt to manage in the circumstances (Askey et al. 2009). When working with carers, it is crucial to challenge our own judgemental thoughts which, unchecked, can lead to staff becoming defensive and attributing blame to the family (Hatfield and Lefley 1987). Staff need instead to develop an understanding about what is going on for each individual and work together towards finding healthy solutions for everyone.

Working with carers is an integral part of the role of mental health professionals but is easily overlooked and often misunderstood (DoH 2002). In Dave's case, we need to differentiate between the actions of his parents and their intentions as they may also feel anxious and worried and the emotional side of caring is often not diminished even though Dave is not with them (DoH 2010). Their concerns may even be exacerbated as they may not perceive that they are able to influence events while Dave is in hospital, and they may also feel excluded from Dave's care. Furthermore, as professionals, we may be accustomed to this environment, but for Dave's parents, it is an unknown and foreboding environment.

Dave's parents often ask staff questions about his unusual beliefs and actions and what he has been doing on the ward and seek to know more about his current programme and treatment. They have complained that some staff do not share information with them.

2   **How do we manage issues of confidentiality in this situation?**

A   Understanding and interpreting issues regarding confidentiality is not straightforward and requires clinical skills and professional judgement (RCP 2004). There is no simple answer, because we must take into account the needs of the service user and the needs of the carer, and each case will be different (DoH 2002). Dave's parents are very keen to understand more about the illness and what is available to help him, yet here it seems some staff perceive this discussion as potentially breaching confidentiality. However, in this decision-making process it is necessary to consider the implications of sharing or not sharing information, because it may have significant implications for the physical and emotional safety and well-being of both service users and carers (DoH 2011).

Furthermore, if carers are not provided with information or included in discussions, it can result in significant, and sometimes highly negative, practical, financial and personal consequences for both the carer and the service user. The implications of not being involved can include an increased sense of separation and further emotional suffering (Kuipers et al. 2010). This can lead to healthcare professionals being viewed as unhelpful, and adversarial relationships develop which cause distress to everyone involved, leading to unfavourable outcomes, which is not beneficial to the service user (Glynn 2006).

Dave tells his nurse that he sometimes feels he has to please his parents and that they still treat him like a child. He feels pressurized to return to his studies but has not been able to say this to them and he is not sure that they should be coming in for the wardround meeting or talking to the staff about him.

3   **What if Dave says no to any contact with his family?**

A   All **codes of professional conduct** for healthcare professions make explicit statements about gaining the consent of service users (NMC 2008; HPC 2007). It is important that we talk to the service user and discuss the benefits and possible challenges of imparting information to carers (RCP 2004). In this case, there may be a role for the staff in supporting Dave to be able to express his feelings to his parents. This will help in negotiating a collaborative plan and will add clarity to the issue of confidentiality in promoting an open dialogue. However, it is also important to be aware that healthcare professionals can talk to carers even if service users do not want confidential information to be shared with the carers as the healthcare professionals can provide general information and work with the carer's needs (Machin 2004). While it is important to work to maintain trust with the service user, listening to the concerns of carers is especially important in the area of risk, as their perspective is an essential component of positive risk management.

> Issues around confidentiality should not be used as a reason for not listening to carers, nor for not discussing fully with service users the need for carers to receive information so that they can continue to support them. Carers should be given sufficient information, in a way they can readily understand, to help them provide care efficiently.
>
> (DoH 2002: 16)

4 **Will working with Dave's parents be of benefit to him?**

A A wealth of evidence has steadily grown regarding the benefits of working with carers over the past four decades (Brown et al. 1972; Falloon et al. 1992; Kuipers et al. 2010). Among the most encouraging outcomes is that by improving carers' knowledge and understanding, they can develop strategies to manage stress and, together with the service user, better manage the challenges of mental illness (Kuipers 2006). Furthermore a carer-focused perspective has influenced national policy and guidance, leading to mental health services being planned and developed to focus on **carer support** and working with carers as a standard consideration of healthcare workers (DoH 2002, 2008, 2011; NICE 2010).

Therefore, there is an expectation that mental health practitioners show empathy for the service user, together with their wider support network, providing information, and practising a recovery-focused approach (Glynn 2006). For the ward staff working with Dave and his family, it was necessary to understand and acknowledge the difficulties they are facing, and to construct a plan which will help them cope with present and future challenges.

Dave's previous comments about his parents' involvement and how he finds it hard to assert himself have made you reflect on the benefits of working with him and his parents, but you are uncertain as to how to proceed.

5 **What approach could you use to work with both clients and carers in routine clinical settings?**

A **Psychosocial interventions (PSI)** is a therapeutic model which encourages the pragmatic use of evidence-based practice to identify and work on improving emotional, social and physical well-being. PSI shares many characteristics with **recovery-based practice**, by focusing on the achievement of personal goals, instilling hope within the family unit, and improving social support (Gamble and Brennan 2006).

A PSI approach addresses the needs of family and carers because they are integral to improving and supporting the well-being of the service user (Kuipers 2006). Ironically, this contrasts with the focus of mental health workers who are trained to focus on the needs of the individual service user. In this case study, some members of the ward team will need to adapt

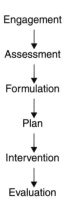

Engagement

↓

Assessment

↓

Formulation

↓

Plan

↓

Intervention

↓

Evaluation

Figure 20.1 The PSI structured approach

their approach to focus to a greater extent on the needs of Dave's parents, which, in turn, will benefit Dave.

PSI places an emphasis on using a structured approach (Figure 20.1) which begins with engagement and assessment, because until the exact issues are known and understood, collaborative and meaningful interventions cannot be planned.

6   **How might we engage with Dave's parents?**

A   Following some discussion with Dave, a meeting was arranged with Dave's parents. Engaging with families and carers is fundamental to subsequent interactions which require us to listen empathically, be non-judgemental and acknowledge distress. By promoting respectful attitudes in this way, we can promote hope and recovery. This part of our work is not about providing answers, but instead developing a positive and collaborative working relationship.

Once a rapport has been established, we can move towards assessment, establishing the views of the carers and gathering information relating to their experiences and interpretations of events (Dixon et al. 2001). The Relatives Assessment Interview (Barrowclough and Tarrier 1997) provides a useful assessment process to understand the impact of caring on the carer physically, emotionally and socially. By looking at these issues with Dave's parents, the health-care worker was able to identify possible areas for collaboration to improve the overall situation for Dave and his parents.

Agenda setting is a technique which can be used each time the healthcare professional meets or communicates with the carers and/or service user. It helps with communication by setting the scene and clarifying boundaries and expectations while also ensuring that we conclude sessions with clarity and identify specific goals and action points for people to achieve. Table 20.1 sets out the framework which can be used for face-to-face meetings or for phone call contact.

Carers often find the experience of caring a significant burden and it is therefore a significant issue which needs consideration. However, the term 'burden' carries negative connotations and it is worth clarifying how carers understand and personally attribute meaning to the way in which burden is evident in their role.

Table 20.1 Agenda setting

1. Introduce yourself if the first time of meeting.
2. Check that the carers/clients are comfortable to proceed.
3. Agree how long the meeting/telephone call will last.
4. Explain and agree the purpose of the meeting/telephone call and that everyone shares the same understanding and expectations.
5. State the expected outcome and ask for everyone's agreement.
6. List the issues to be discussed and agree the order of priority.
7. Ask if anybody wants to include anything else.
8. Go through the order of the agenda.
9. Conduct the meeting in accordance with the agenda.
10. Use the agenda to review and evaluate the meeting/interaction.

The concept of burden has been much discussed in the literature for many years and can be seen as composed of two dimensions: objective and subjective. More recently much of the literature pertaining to burden has attempted to identify associated factors that mental health workers need to consider, and there are many factors which will vary between individual families (Shah et al. 2010). These can be difficult issues to discuss and we may need to consider that the work could involve a number of sessions/contacts (NICE 2010).

THE CONCEPT OF BURDEN

- *Objective burden* relates to that which exists externally and can be observed by others. This includes physical care, finance, poor living conditions and overcrowding.
- *Subjective burden* is less tangible and viewed as personal, internal feelings such as guilt, shame, worry, attitudes, perceptions of experiences, and worries.

Factors which we need to consider include:

- effect on carers of the behaviour of a person with a mental health problem;
- effect of caring on carer's own health;
- carers' lack of social engagement due to social isolation; reduced contact with family and friends; fear of stigma;
- implications for finances and employment;
- relationships within the wider family network;
- other relatives and the offering or adoption of inappropriate/unhelpful advice;
- children and their care or providing care to the person with a mental health problem;
- perceived helpfulness/unhelpfulness of mental health services;
- carers' knowledge and adjustment to mental health problem.

PSI for carers sets out to understand the individual carer's experiences, attitudes and beliefs and burden, before deciding together with them on a plan of interventions. The overall aim of PSI is to provide short-term and importantly long-term, flexible strategies for coping.

OUTCOME OF ASSESSMENT

Dave's parents were feeling emotionally and physically exhausted. They said that they hadn't slept properly in weeks and were concerned that Dave might hurt himself or someone else, but they struggle to talk openly with Dave. They worry about Dave's future and his mum is considering giving up work to look after him, but his dad thinks Dave should be more independent. They do not know what to say to family and friends and have become isolated. They feel that they are perceived as a problem and feel guilty that they have in some way contributed to Dave's 'breakdown'. Both parents want to know more about what is wrong with Dave and the treatments that are available but feel that they never get a direct answer, which causes them frustration and anguish.

7   **What are the main interventions that could be helpful for Dave and his parents?**

A   From the outcome of the assessment, our plan could include the use of three interventions that would be of benefit in addressing both psychological and practical issues (Mueser 2003). These will help Dave's parents to understand more about Dave's mental health problem and assist with improving their knowledge of what may be helpful. These three interventions are: (1) techniques for helping to solve everyday problems; (2) improve dialogue with Dave; and (3) improve communication with services. Combining these approaches will work towards establishing helpful coping strategies which the evidence suggests can reduce the risk of relapse (Pharoah et al. 2006) (Table 20.2).

Table 20.2 Useful interventions

Coping approach	Description
Psycho-education	Psycho-education combines emotional support with knowledge development in order for people to make sense of the situations they find themselves in and the experiences they have. This is clearly something that Dave's parents have been looking for. It is not designed to provide all the answers but to open up discussion, dispel myths and present new ways of thinking and alternative ways of doing things (DoH 2002)
Problem solving	Problem solving aims to develop confidence and the ability to make helpful and informed choices. It also ameliorates the emotional burden of caring. While the difficult emotions associated with the burden of caring will not be eradicated, using this approach permits the identification of other workable possibilities. Therefore, this intervention is not simply about short-term gains, but developing a structured, objective and less emotive way of managing difficulties (Falloon et al. 1984; Mueser 2003).

Among the options which might be included are setting realistic and achievable goals for Dave to resume his studies or looking at his options for the future

Communication skills   Having regular meetings involving Dave and his parents allows staff to promote and model alternative, helpful and positive ways of communicating. This ensures clarity, reduces distress and effectively manages difficult or challenging situations effectively (Askey et al. 2009; Kuipers 2006)

EVALUATION

Evaluation needs to be part of an ongoing process and links back to agenda setting by taking everyone's views into account and recognizing achievements, while identifying issues that still need further work and enhancing collaboration and a sense of personal participation.

In the months that followed, through regular family meetings Dave was able to make important steps towards his recovery with the support of his parents and the mental health team (Table 20.3).

Over time, the whole family were able to understand that by developing knowledge and skills through having open and honest communication, they could all focus on having a healthy lifestyle and use more effective ways of coping. This promoted well-being for everybody.

Table 20.3 Dave's recovery progress

	Dave	*Mum and Dad*
Communication	Dave was able to understand and appreciate why his parents were so protective, but was able to express how this made him feel	Mum and Dad gained insight into how Dave felt and understood how their attempts to help were sometimes misunderstood
Psycho-education	Increased awareness of early warning signs and coping strategies	Developed knowledge of medication and treatment and accessing carers' support
Problem solving	Developed a plan for returning to college and maintained well-being through physical exercise and healthy routines	Increased confidence in Dave's recovery allowed parents to resume their own roles and activities

CONCLUSION

Through effective, objective, and evidence-based engagement with Dave's family, we can see that we are able to develop helpful and productive relationships that can be of benefit to Dave, his family and our services. Working together gives us the opportunity to learn from each other; this is a powerful and practical strategy to mediate and effectively manage the potentially destructive consequences of psychological distress. Therefore, while this work represents a challenge for mental health workers, it is also an area of great promise that needs to be practised, promoted and progressed in order to firmly establish recovery-based approaches for all those involved.

REFERENCES

Askey, R. et al. (2009) What do carers of people with psychosis need from mental health services? Exploring the views of carers, service users and professionals. *Journal of Family Therapy*, 31(3): 310–31.

Barrowclough, C. and Tarrier, N. (1997) *Families of Schizophrenic Patients: Cognitive Behavioural Intervention*. Cheltenham: Stanley Thornes.

Brown, G., Birley, J. and Wing, J. (1972) Influence of family life on the course of schizophrenic disorders: a replication, *British Journal of Psychiatry*, 121: 241–58.

Dixon, L. et al. (2001) Evidence-based practices for services to families of people with psychiatric disabilities, *Psychiatric Services*, 52: 903–10.

DoH (Department of Health) (2002) *Developing Services for Carers and Families of People with Mental Illness*. London: DoH.

DoH (Department of Health) (2008) *Refocusing the Care Programme Approach*. London: DoH.

DoH (Department of Health) (2010) *Recognised, Valued and Supported: Next Steps for the Carers Strategy*. London: DoH.

DoH (Department of Health) (2011) *No Health Without Mental Health*. London: DoH.

Falloon, I.R.H., Boyd, J.L. and McGill, C. (1984) *Family Care of Schizophrenia*. London: Guilford Press.

Falloon, I.R.H., Jeffrey, M., Boyd, L., McGill, C., Razani, J., Moss, H., and Gilderman, A. (1992) Family management in the prevention of morbidity in schizophrenia: social outcome of a two-year longitudinal study, *Psychological Medicine*, 17: 59–66.

Gamble, C. and Brennan, G. (2006) *Working with Serious Mental Illness*. London: Ballière Tindall.

Glynn, S. (2006) The potential impact of the recovery movement on family interventions for schizophrenia: opportunities and obstacles, *Schizophrenia Bulletin*, 32(3): 451–63.

Hatfield, A. and Lefley, P. (1987) *Families of the Mentally Ill: Coping and Adaptation*. London: Guilford Press.

HPC (Health Professions Council) (2007) *Standards of Performance, Conduct and Ethics*. London: HPC.

Kuipers, E. (2006) Family interventions in schizophrenia: evidence for efficacy and proposed mechanisms of change, *Journal of Family Therapy*, 28(1): 73–80.

Kuipers, E., Onwumere, J. and Bebbington, P. (2010) Cognitive model of caregiving in psychosis, *British Journal of Psychiatry*, 19(6): 259–65.

Machin, G. (2004) Carers and confidentiality: law and good practice, paper presented to Carers' Council Conference, Edwinstowe, 23 April 2004.

Mueser, K. (2003) *Family Services for Severe Mental Illness*. Dartmouth, NH: Dartmouth Psychiatric Research Center Department of Psychiatry, Dartmouth Medical School.

NICE (National Institute of Health and Clinical Excellence) (2010) *Quick Reference Guide to Schizophrenia*. Clinical Guideline 82. London: NICE.

NMC (Nursing and Midwifery Council) (2008) *The Code: Standards of Conduct, Performance and Ethics for Nurses and Midwifes*. London: NMC.

Pharoah, F., Mari, J., Rathbone, J. and Wong, W. (2006) Family intervention for schizophrenia, *Cochrane Database of Systematic Reviews*, 2006(4).

Pilling, S., Bebbington, P., Kuipers, E., Garety, P., Geddes, J., Orbach, G., et al. (2002) Psychological treatments in schizophrenia: I. Meta-analysis of family intervention and cognitive behaviour therapy, *Psychological Medicine*, 32(5): 763–82.

RCP (Royal College of Psychiatrists) (2004) *Carers and Confidentiality in Mental Health: Issues Involved in Information Sharing*. Carers and Confidentiality leaflet. Available at: http://www.partnersincare.co.uk_download campaign materials (accessed 3 November 2011).

Shah, A., Wadoo, O. and Latoo, J. (2010) Psychological distress in carers of people with mental disorders, *British Journal of Medical Practitioners*, 3(3): 327.

Zubin, J. and Spring, B. (1977) Vulnerability: a new view on schizophrenia, *Journal of Abnormal Psychology*, 86: 103–26.

James is 19 years old and lives on the outskirts of a small town with his parents and two younger sisters, Emily, who is 11, and Louise, who is 15. Their parents own their business but it is struggling, and James has been working part-time in the family business while saving money to go to college, and has been in a relationship with Sophie whom he met at school for a number of years. They had been very happy together and planned to marry next year. However, Sophie ended the relationship six months ago because she said that James had become distant and was drinking much more, but they are still friends.

James's family have noticed that over the last few months he has been staying in his room and not getting dressed; he has refused to join the family for meals and is eating prepackaged food. James is also irritable when anyone speaks to him and drinks several cans of strong lager a day. One afternoon Louise told James that she is worried about him as she has seen comments which he has posted on Facebook and which scared her and Emily. James became angry and shouted at Louise, pushing past her to run out of the house. When he returned home much later, he looked dishevelled, tearful and after some discussion was persuaded by his mum to go and see the family G P.

When James went to see his G P, he told the doctor that he is scared and does not understand what is happening to him. James said that he is finding it difficult to concentrate because the government is reading his mind and communicating with him by Twitter, and trying to control him by broadcasting subliminal messages through Facebook on his laptop, as a result of which he has thrown out the laptop and his iPhone to stop the messages. The G P suggested that James see a psychiatrist.

James and his mum attended an appointment with a psychiatrist and James asked to see the psychiatrist on his own. The psychiatrist asked James a number of questions about his past and what he was experiencing. James looked very distracted and kept repeating the psychiatrist's questions, forgetting what he had said and giving very brief answers. He kept looking around the room, especially at the light switch and asked the psychiatrist if he was being videoed. The psychiatrist tells James that what is happening to him is a psychotic episode of schizophrenia.

1   **How might you identify if someone is experiencing schizophrenia?**

A   The psychiatrist asked a number of questions to find out what had happened to James in the past. For example, how long he had been experiencing problems, and how he is feeling at the present. It is important to establish that what is happening to James is a disruption to his usual functioning, and has been occurring for at least four weeks in duration (Norman and Ryrie 2009).

Schizophrenia is a major psychiatric disorder, or cluster of disorders affecting about 1 per cent of men and women across all cultures, and usually develops between the ages of 16 and

30 years old (NIMH 2009); it is diagnosed using the International Classification of Diseases (ICD-10). Negative perceptions caused by fear and mistaken cultural stereotypes mean schizophrenia is often the subject of stigma and labelling, which makes adjusting to this diagnosis very difficult for James, his family and friends. Being diagnosed with schizophrenia can lead to social exclusion, the loss of friends and social opportunities, difficulties with relationships and an increased chance of suicide (NICE 2009). Therefore it is important to establish that any diagnosis of schizophrenia is correct for a person such as James, and because of this it is unusual for a diagnosis to be given on a first presentation, and other investigations such as blood and urine tests need to be considered to rule out any other possible factors or causes.

James appears to have been experiencing difficulties for some time, has been frightened about what is happening to him and has hidden this from his family until it is no longer possible to do so. These difficulties include a range of symptoms that are affecting all aspects of him as a person, including his behaviour, cognitions and perceptions.

The signs and symptoms of schizophrenia are often divided into two broad categories which are called positive symptoms and negative symptoms. Positive symptoms are psychotic features which exaggerate the normal perceptions of the individual, and can include hallucinations, thought disorders and **delusions**. In contrast, negative symptoms are a reduction in the normal experience of the individual. These often develop more slowly, and are harder to recognize, especially in younger people. Negative symptoms often resemble depression and affect normal moods and behaviours and can cause significant distress, as they can be misinterpreted particularly in younger adults and adolescents as laziness, or regarded as part of teenage development. Among negative symptoms are: **anhedonia**, **cognitive difficulties**, social withdrawal and difficulties in planning and sustaining activities.

An individual's behaviour may be affected as a consequence of the experience of both positive and negative symptoms. For example, James threw away his laptop because he thought it was controlling his thoughts, and he is avoiding people because he is feeling scared and trying to protect his family from what is happening to him (Norman and Ryrie 2009). Agitated and repetitive movements can also be experienced with schizophrenia (NIMH 2009), or as a potentially unwanted side effect from medication, and need further investigation.

2 **Concerning James's behaviour and the content of his discussion with the GP and psychiatrist, what possible positive and negative symptoms of schizophrenia could he be experiencing? And how might these affect his behaviour?**

A Positive symptoms that James is experiencing are:

- James is hearing voices coming from his laptop, which could be auditory hallucinations or voices.
- James has said that the government is communicating to him by Twitter on to his laptop, and through his iPhone, which is an example of a **thought disorder (ideas of reference)**.
- James believes people are talking about him, which could be an example of a **persecutory delusion**, or might be grounded in fact, and needs further investigation.
- James believes the government is trying to control him, which could be an example of passivity phenomena.

Negative symptoms which James is experiencing are:

- James is not going out and is staying in his room and drinking more than usual. Some people who hear voices use alcohol or other drugs to self-medicate and ease the distress caused by their illness. In James's case, his increased use of alcohol might represent a coping mechanism in response to the intensification of his symptoms.
- James is having difficulties concentrating and appears distracted, giving brief answers; he is repeating the same sentence and losing the thread of the conversation, which could be evidence of cognitive difficulties.
- His girlfriend, Sophie, has described his personality as altered and that he is not the same as before.

His behaviour is altered:

- James is looking around the room and asking if he is being videoed; this could be because he is experiencing a persecutory delusion.
- James has been throwing out his electronic devices due to his thought disorder.
- James is not eating with the family and is buying his own food which could be an example of paranoia as he may feel the food is poisoned or interfered with in some way and this needs further exploration with James.
- James has become more irritable in mood and has a low threshold for anger.

3 **What are the possible causes (aetiology) of schizophrenia?**

 Schizophrenia is thought to be an interaction between genetics and environmental factors (Kyriakopoulos and Frangou 2007) and although there have been many explanations suggested, there is still no definitive agreed cause.

However, it is generally thought that it is determined by a number of genes (polygenic), and that these susceptible genes interact with environmental factors (Mueser and McGurk 2004). Therefore, it is believed that there is a high genetic factor associated with schizophrenia with it being believed to be inherited (Kyriakopoulos and Frangou 2007). For example, there is a 50 per cent chance of a child being diagnosed with schizophrenia when both parents are affected (Mueser and McGurk 2004).

However, environmental factors are also believed to contribute to schizophrenia and theories regarding this can be divided into biological and sociodemographic.

- Biological factors can occur during pregnancy, for example, maternal influenza, rubella, malnutrition and complications during labour such as **hypoxia** (Mueser and McGurk 2004).
- With regard to sociodemographic factors, there are two explanatory theories. The first of these is the social causation theory which suggests that life is more stressful for those in the lower socioeconomic groups, and this, combined with a genetic vulnerability, can give rise to the development of schizophrenia. The downward social drift theory suggests that the combination of experiencing severe and enduring mental illness, together with stigma and unemployment, leads to a decline in people's prospects and circumstances and forces them into poverty and social exclusion. It has also been discovered that there is an increased prevalence of schizophrenia in urban areas rather than rural areas, and within some ethnic

minority groups, which is believed to be due to the interaction between the stress of being a minority group and genetic vulnerability (Mueser and McGurk 2004).

There is also thought to be a link between drug use and schizophrenia. While it is unclear whether it causes schizophrenia, there is general agreement that drug use increases the risk of developing schizophrenia (Arendt et al. 2005).

Schizophrenia can progress through three stages. These are not distinct or separate stages, and are known as the **premorbid stage**, the **prodromal stage** and then the experience of psychosis. The prodromal stage can be between 1–5 years in duration and an individual may experience some depression, anxiety and sleep problems in those years before the psychotic episode develops (Freudenreich, et al. 2007).

The psychiatrist asked James a number of questions about his family and childhood development to discover if there were any members of the family with a mental health problem to establish any genetic vulnerability. The psychiatrist asked James about how much alcohol he drank each day and whether he has taken any drugs. James said he drank because it helps him feel calm but he did not take any other drugs. The psychiatrist also asked questions about his birth, childhood and any events in his life that might indicate any environmental or developmental factors, for example, difficulties at school, stressful experiences, to gain an insight into any influential environmental factors. James is hoping to go to college, and has an interview in a few weeks time. When James was a teenager, he found it difficult to attend school and often got into trouble; he said he found school boring and could not be bothered to go. He also got into fights as he believed other school kids were calling him names.

When the psychiatrist told James that he had schizophrenia, he became very distressed. He said that someone had been putting drugs into his water and this was what was causing the problem. A urine test was used to see if there were any drugs in his system which produced a negative result. James then tried to leave the consulting room so his mum came in to try to comfort James and find out what was happening, but James refused to talk to her and left. His mum was upset and talked to the psychiatrist, explaining that she had been worried about James for some time. He had become increasingly withdrawn, and was not going out with his friends. His mum had been worried that James might be taking drugs or that he was worried about the family business and that this might be causing his strange behaviour.

Later during the evening James returned home drunk. His mum persuaded James to tell her what was wrong, but he was upset and distant and said that he wished he were dead, which upset her. James's mum didn't know how to help James, and when speaking to her husband said that she felt she was losing her son, and that the failure of the business might be adding to James's mental health problems, and she was worried about his future and what would happen to him. She has heard that people with schizophrenia get locked up and given all kinds of medications and are never the same again.

4   How can the family be supported in coming to terms with the diagnosis James has been given?

A   The family will all need time to adjust to what is happening to James. His mum will be given the offer of a **carers assessment**; Emily and Louise's needs will also need to be assessed. The family will be provided with details of any local support groups and voluntary organizations and given help in accessing these services. It is important to involve the family in the negotiation and management of the care provided for James to give him the best outcome and to preserve the family as a support network which is important to James and his recovery (NICE 2009).

5 **What support and treatment are available for James?**

A James will need time to come to terms with his diagnosis, and the many losses that he might experience. These are primary losses brought on by schizophrenia, for example, the impairment of cognitive and emotional functioning, and also secondary losses, such as independence and the loss of vocation, status, and self-esteem (Wittmann and Keshaven 2007).

James was hoping to go to college but now it might not be possible at this time and will be more difficult in the future. He is experiencing a number of cognitive difficulties and thought disorders that will disrupt his ability to concentrate and function, and will affect his career choices and his confidence. James is already experiencing difficulties within his familial relationships, has lost contact with his friends, and his long-term relationship has ended. This is reducing his social support, leading to isolation and may further reduce his ability to function socially.

The NICE guidelines for schizophrenia (2009) give the best practice for supporting James and his family:

- James may need the support of a community mental health team. The team will appoint a lead professional or a **care coordinator**. This could be a nurse, occupational therapist, or a social worker and depends upon what James's needs are as to which healthcare professional is best able to offer person-centred support for James (DoH 2007).
- His care coordinator will take time to get to know James and to offer him a comprehensive multi-disciplinary assessment of psychiatric, psychological and physical health. The assessment will also consider any issues that James may have regarding accommodation, culture, economic status and education, drugs history, quality of life, responsibility for children, risks of harm to self and others, sexual health and social networks.
- James is experiencing a lot of distress at the moment, and might not feel ready to think about employment, education or occupational needs. When James is ready, it is important that these needs are considered for his recovery, and his care coordinator will work alongside him and local stakeholders to enable James to access local employment and educational opportunities.
- James will be offered **antipsychotic medication** to help manage his experiences. It is important to agree the choice of drug with James, by giving him information on the potential side effects and benefits of antipsychotic medication, and for him to feel able to discuss his concerns, be involved in his care, and willing to take medication which is suited to his needs (NICE 2009).
- James's physical health will be monitored by his GP.
- James may be offered psychological therapies, such as cognitive behavioural therapy (CBT), which can be started at either the acute phase or later.
- James may need a period of time in hospital or with intensive support to help him through this initial acute phase; this should be considered carefully, by looking at all the information on risks, whether he needs to go to an in-patient setting or if he can be supported at home.
- James will be encouraged and involved in developing a crisis management plan based on understanding any early warning signs that James or his family recognize, for example,

when James begins to stay in his room and eat prepackaged food, this might indicate that he is beginning to experience some thought disorder again.

James has experienced a severe psychotic episode that has led to a diagnosis of schizophrenia; this is a severe and enduring mental illness that is likely to continue to affect James to some extent in his daily life. Recovery for each person is an individual journey and the professionals involved with James will focus on empowering James to self-manage his experience by developing his own unique strategies to maintain his well-being and to support James in achieving his maximum potential. James has a supportive family, and as a family they are all working towards recovery for James. When his symptoms are less intrusive, James is returning to work to continue to save money towards attending a college course and commencing his career.

REFERENCES

Arendt, M. et al. (2005) Cannabis induced psychosis and subsequent schizophrenia, *British Journal of Psychiatry*, 187: 510–15.

DoH (Department of Health) (2007) *New Ways of Working for Everyone: Best Practice Implementation Guide*. Available at: http://www.dh.gov.uk/prod_consum_dh/groups/dh_digitalassets/@dh/@en/documents/digitalasset/dh_079106.pdf (accessed 6 February 2011).

DoH (Department of Health) (2008) *Reviewing the Care Programme Approach*. Available at: http://www.dh.gov.uk/en/Publicationsandstatistics/Publications/PublicationsPolicyAndGuidance/DH_083647 (accessed 6 February 2011).

Freudenreich, O., Holt, D.J., Cather, C. and Goff, D.C. (2007) The evaluation and management of patients with first-episode schizophrenia: a selective, clinical review of diagnosis, treatment and prognosis, *Harvard Review of Psychiatry*, 15: 189–211.

Galbraith, A., Bullock, S., Manias, E., Hunt, B. and Richards, A. (2002) *Fundamentals of Pharmacology, An Applied Approach for Nursing and Health*. 2nd edn. Harlow: Pearson Education.

Kyriakopoulos, M. and Frangou, S. (2007) Pathophysiology of early onset schizophrenia, *International Review of Psychiatry*, 19(4): 315–24.

Mueser, K.T. and McGurk, S.R. (2004) Schizophrenia, *The Lancet*, 363: 2063–72.

NICE (National Institute of Health and Clinical Excellence) (2009) *Medicines Adherence: Quick Reference Guide*. Available at: http://www.nice.org.uk/nicemedia/live/11766/42891/42891.pdf (accessed 6 February 2011).

NIMH (National Institute of Mental Health) (2009) *Schizophrenia*. Available at: http://www.nimh.nih.gov/health/publications/schizophrenia/schizophrenia-booket-2009.pdf (accessed 8 June 2011).

Norman, I. and Ryrie, I. (eds) (2009) *The Art and Science of Mental Health Nursing*, 2nd edn. Maidenhead: McGraw-Hill.

Wittmann, D. and Keshaven, M. (2007) Grief and mourning in schizophrenia, *Psychiatry*, 70(2): 154–66.

Caring for a person with bipolar disorder
Geoffrey Amoateng

Marion is in her mid-fifties and has had a long history of bipolar affective disorder for much of her adult life. When growing up Marion had a happy childhood, as an only child living with her supportive and caring parents in a wealthy neighbourhood. Marion was a bright student who excelled at school, achieved good grades and then left home to study at a prestigious university. However, at this point in her life she began to experience the onset of bipolar disorder, and eventually became too unwell to continue with her course.

Marion now lives in a warden-controlled flat. She has never married, although has had some close relationships, and has just a few friends preferring to isolate herself and avoid being in company. Marion keeps her flat tidy and among her interests and activities she watches soap operas on television, regularly attends bingo and smokes a few cigarettes each day. Over the years Marion has had numerous in-patient admissions, some of which have been against her will and compulsory under the Mental Health Act (1983). She has bad memories of being unwell and associates these unpleasant experiences with involvement with the mental health services. Her last admission was reluctantly informal and occurred nine years ago after she became low in mood following the death of her cat.

Since her last admission, Marion's mental state has been fairly stable; she has remained on the same medication, and regularly attended appointments with her G P, with whom she has a good relationship, to monitor her mood.

After a minor operation at a local hospital, Marion's friends noticed a significant change in her mood. In contrast with her usual quiet manner, she became talkative, bought everyone gifts and told her friends that she had inherited money from a long-lost relative whom she had never mentioned previously. Marion was restless and agitated, and kept her neighbours awake at night by playing Christmas carols, even though it was not that time of year. Marion was uncharacteristically loud in her tone of voice and flirted with the warden and her G P.

Marion was offered an admission to an adult mental health ward by her G P to review her medication. However, the local mental health Trust has a policy of in-patient admissions being 'gate kept' by the Crisis Resolution and Home Treatment (C R H T) team, who are based in the community. Marion was disappointed that she had become unwell again, and reluctantly agreed to be referred to the C R H T team.

1 **What is bipolar disorder?**

A Bipolar disorder is characterized by the occurrence of at least one episode of **mania** or **hypomania**, and the person usually also experiences further recurrent major depressive episodes (American Psychiatric Association 2000; World Health Organization 1992). Mania or hypomania is not simply being a little over-excited, but instead a period of persistently elevated mood, consisting of euphoria and expansive goodwill, but also negative emotions such as fear, irritability and anger.

In contrast, a hypomanic episode is less pronounced than mania, and while not sufficiently severe to interrupt daily life, is nevertheless manifest in a number of ways, which include:

- elevated mood;
- increased activity;
- perceived reduced need for sleep;
- grandiose ideas;
- racing thoughts.

Generally, there are perceived to be two levels of bipolar disorder:

- Bipolar I: refers to people who are experiencing mania but not hypomania.
- Bipolar II: pertains to people experiencing hypomania and features of depression but not mania.

There is an overlap between depression and bipolar disorder. Young and MacPherson (2011) suggest that quite often people with bipolar disorder have had multiple episodes of major depression before their first experience of mania and people with hypomania and depression are commonly said to have bipolar II disorder (NICE 2010). Many of the features of bipolar disorder are also consistent with those experienced in depression.

Manic episodes usually begin abruptly and can last for between 2 weeks and 4–5 months, although care and treatment may be initiated sooner where the person is experiencing bipolar disorder type I, due to the severity of the person's distress, and the consideration of risk for the person and others.

The features of bipolar disorder include a range of changes in emotion, cognition, behaviour and physical functioning (Table 22.1). Once known as **manic depression**, it is now more commonly referred to as bipolar disorder, which reflects the severe swings in mood which the person experiences. These mood swings are far beyond what most of us usually experience in our day-to-day life where our frame of mind can vary but instead range from feeling extremely low or intense depression and despair, to feelings of elation and happiness or irritability, and mania and depression may alternate with one another in mood cycles.

While bipolar disorder is characterized by extremes of mood, other features are also often evident which resemble other mental health problems. For example, some people experience symptoms of psychosis, such as seeing or hearing things which other people do not, in the form of visual or auditory hallucinations, or express strange or unusual beliefs which other people do not share, which are referred to as delusions. The person may also continually feel tired, have a pervasive low mood, lack pleasure in things which they used to enjoy and have sleep problems and frequent thoughts of suicide or self-harm, which are all commonly experienced in depression.

About 1–2 per cent of the general population is diagnosed with bipolar disorder, and a roughly equal number of men and women (American Psychiatric Association 2000). While it can affect people of any age, from children to older adults, as with Marion, it often develops in late adolescence or early adulthood, with at least half of all cases starting before the age of 25 (Kessler et al. 2003). Although some people will experience individual episodes and feel

Table 22.1 Signs and symptoms of manic/hypomanic episodes

Emotional changes	Cognitive changes	Behavioural changes	Physical changes
Mood swings between euphoria (excessively high) and elation to anger and irritability	Racing thoughts	Dramatic mannerisms, flamboyant dress and make-up	Full of energy, does not tire easily
Switches of affect from happy to depressed and hostile	Distractible	Increase in goal-directed activity	Extreme motor activity leading to exhaustion
Uncritical self-confidence	Rapid and loud speech that is difficult to interrupt	Increase in goal-directed activity	Insomnia with decreased need for sleep
Wish to be gratified in whatever the person does	Flight of ideas and poor judgement	Intrusive, demanding, domineering and sometimes aggressive	Weight loss/gain or changes in appetite
Restlessness and chronic fatigue	Impaired judgement	Resists efforts to treat	Lack of attention to personal hygiene, appearance and general health
Lack of concentration	Ideas of reference, delusions and hallucinations	Dislikes having wishes thwarted	
	Impulsive	Aggressive behaviour	
	Acts in sexual ways that are unusual for the person, e.g. hypersexuality	Talking very fast	

Source: Barker (2003: 282).

well for the rest of the time, others will not get better fully between episodes or, like Marion, experience lost opportunities in work, education and relationships, but nevertheless manage some level of equilibrium and quality of life.

2 **What causes bipolar disorder?**

A The causes of bipolar disorder are not well understood. Some research suggests that it runs in families, and has more to do with genes than upbringing (Barker 2009). However, some people will experience bipolar disorder without there being a pre-existent family history. Yet the notion that there is a physiological explanation gains support from the effectiveness of medication, such as **lithium** and anti-convulsants, which it is believed remedy problems with the function of the nerves in the brain which cause bipolar disorder. Other research suggests there is a different physical cause for bipolar disorder in the form of disturbances in the endocrine system which controls hormones (Healy 2002).

However, there is also much research suggesting that there are a range of other factors active in triggering bipolar disorder. According to Barker (2009), these include:

- stress;
- environment;
- social factors;
- sleep disturbance;
- physical illness.

Consistent with these findings, a person who first experiences bipolar disorder in later life is more likely to be associated with co-morbid physical disorders (Duffy et al. 2009).

3   **How do you recognize bipolar disorder?**

A   Recognizing bipolar disorder in adults, particularly those who have not experienced it before, can be difficult and many people have periods of considerable psychological and social upheaval before it is confirmed that they are experiencing this problem. A person with bipolar disorder might display some of the characteristics identified in Table 22.1.

4   **Can you identify which features of Marion's behaviour might indicate a recurrence of her bipolar disorder?**

A   The features which she is displaying, and that might indicate a recurrence of bipolar disorder for Marion are:

- marked change in mood;
- talkative;
- playing her music very loud at night and keeping neighbours awake;
- restlessness;
- agitation;
- her belief about inheriting money from a relative which she had not mentioned before may be mistaken;
- impulsive buying of gifts;
- disinhibition by flirting with the warden and her GP.

5   **Until very recently Marion's mental state has been fairly stable for several years and she has remained on the same medication. What is the recommended treatment for bipolar disorder?**

A   Most people living in the community who experience bipolar disorder will automatically go to see their family doctor who may make a referral to a psychiatrist to discuss the treatments which are available. There are two objectives for treatment: (1) stopping the episode of depression or mania; and (2) minimizing the risk of relapse where this has been a recurrent problem. Often people will experience ongoing episodes of acute depression and bipolar disorder, and in this situation the goal is to reduce the severity and ensure that the person can access help and support rapidly.

A variety of treatments are available, ranging from medication, to talking treatments such as cognitive behavioural therapy (CBT), and these can be carried out in an in-patient hospital setting, if the person is acutely unwell and presents a high level of risk to themselves or others, or is vulnerable, or in the community (Norman and Ryrie 2009).

Increasingly mental health services have focused on working with people in their own homes. The C R H T to which Marion has been referred is an example of the range of community-based mental health services introduced as a result of the *National Service Framework for Mental Health* (DoH 1999), which aimed to make mental health services more accessible and flexible to the needs of people with mental health problems. An advantage of community-based mental health services in the case of Marion is that being supported in the home environment avoids the potential distress of being required to go into hospital, of which she has unpleasant memories concerning her past experiences, but which would also necessitate reorientation to her home environment after discharge from the in-patient services.

TREATMENT FOR BIPOLAR DISORDER

Medication

Almost everyone who has bipolar disorder will be offered medication, and many people such as Marion find that this helps reduce the severity of their symptoms, stabilize mood and can prevent relapse. However, medication should be seen as part of a range of care planned interventions, which take account of the individual's needs, preferences and wishes.

Differences in response to medication often determine the preferred choice of drug. For example, the person may experience unwanted changes, such as uncomfortable side effects. Furthermore, precautions need to be considered, which relate to, for example, age, gender, health issues or contraindications with other medications which are being taken that might make it unsuitable to be prescribed a particular drug. For example, the teratogenic and neuro-behavioural toxicity associated with valproate severely limits its use in women of child-bearing age.

Although medication cannot cure bipolar disorder, and it is generally agreed that effective treatment should include both medication and psychotherapy, it still performs an important role in supporting people to maintain quality of life (Sachs et al. 2000). Table 22.2 identifies common medications used in the treatment of bipolar disorder.

Table 22.2 Medication used in the treatment of bipolar disorder

Drug name	Precautions	Special measures	Side effects
Lithium – lithium carbonate, (Camcolit, Liskonum), and lithium citrate (Li-Liquid, Priadel)	• Lithium is not suitable for children • A person who is on lithium medication will require regular blood tests to make sure that the level of	• Often prescribed for mania • The type of lithium taken is not relevant so long as one keeps to the same one at each point in time	• Weight gain • Oedema • Renal impairment • Thirst • Gastro-intestinal disturbances (anorexia, vomiting, and diarrhoea) and tremor • Muscle weakness

(Continued overleaf)

Table 22.2 Continued

Drug name	Precautions	Special measures	Side effects
	lithium in his or her blood is safe and effective (every 3 months on stabilized regimens) • Measure renal function and thyroid function every 6–12 months	• It is important for one to maintain steady salt and water levels as far as possible when taking lithium medication • Long-term use is potentially toxic to the thyroid gland and the kidneys, and their function should be checked regularly during treatment	
Anticonvulsant: Semi-sodium valproate (Depakote). Valproate is available in other forms, including sodium valproate and valproic acid	• Monitor liver function before treatment during first 6 months	• The active element in all formulations is the valproate and is the generic term used by most people	• Nausea • Weight gain • Gastric irritation • Diarrhoea • Increased alertness • Aggression • Drowsiness • Confusion • Vomiting
Antidepressants: Carbamazepine (Tegretol)	Carbamazepine may be used for the prophylaxis of bipolar disorder	• Patients should be reviewed every 1–2 weeks at the start of anti-depressant treatment	• Confusion and agitation • Nausea and vomiting • Dizziness • Diarrhoea • Headaches • Leucopenia and other blood disorders
Lamotrigine (Lamictal)	• Closely monitor and withdraw if rash, fever or other signs of hypersensitivity • Avoid abrupt withdrawal at beginning of treatment. (See the British National Formulary for more information)	• Lamotrigine has anti-depressant effects and is licensed for the prevention of depressive episodes in bipolar disorder	• Skin rashes • Hyper-sensitivity syndrome • Nausea • Vomiting • Diarrhoea

Antipsychotics:
Olanzapine
(Zyprexa),
Quetiapine
(Seroquel),
Risperidone
(Risperdal) and
Aripiprazole
(Abilify).
Haloperidol
(Haldol, Dozic,
Serenace) or
Chlorpromazine
(Largactil).

- Any antipsychotic drugs used should be licensed for the treatment of mania in the United Kingdom and may be taken at the same time as an anticonvulsant or lithium
- Please see the Guideline for treatment and management of bipolar disorder (www.nice.org.uk/guideline)

The management of acute manic and hypomanic episodes depends on the severity of symptoms and whether patients are currently taking anti-manic drugs

- Extrapyramidal symptoms like Parkinsonian disease (including tremor)
- Akathisia (restlessness), which occurs after large initial doses and may resemble an exacerbation of the condition being treated
- Drowsiness, agitation, excitement and insomnia, headaches and dizziness

Electroconvulsive
therapy (ECT)
(In NHS hospitals
this is used in the
treatment of severe
manic and
depressive
episodes.)

- This is recommended for patients only when it is deemed to achieve rapid and short-term improvement of severe symptoms after an adequate trial of other treatment options has proven ineffective and/or when the condition is considered to be potentially life-threatening, in individuals with severe depressive illness, catatonia, and a prolonged or severe manic episode.

Psychotherapeutic interventions

The use of talking therapies, for example, cognitive behavioural therapy (CBT) is well recognized as helping to reduce both the potential and extent of relapse for people with bipolar disorder. CBT aims to help people to identify problems and overcome emotional difficulties, and is a practical talking treatment, but also relies on the person making changes to their behaviour and focusing on changing negative thought patterns which are often associated with bipolar disorder. When used together with medication, many people with bipolar disorder find these combined treatments to be a great help. It is suggested that CBT reduces residual symptoms and enhances the effect of lithium in preventing relapse (Fava et al. 2002; Norman and Ryrie 2009).

Other talking therapy options such as counselling, psychotherapy or sessions with a psychologist can also help people with bipolar disorder understand and challenge their feelings. Also these therapies permit the person to facilitate change in the way they think and experience and manage their emotions by offering an opportunity to talk about the stressful experience of bipolar disorder and develop better coping mechanisms.

The nurse with the CRHT conducted a mental state assessment. As Marion has had previous compulsory in-patient admissions, she has felt reluctant to engage with services due to associating these with her periods of mental ill-health but also unfortunately, out of necessity, the loss of her liberty. It was important to create a therapeutic, person-centred rapport with her, based on acceptance, genuineness, empathy and intuition in order to build a trusting understanding (Watkins 2007).

The assessment took the form of a conversation and permitted Marion to tell her story rather than a series of questions based on the documentation, or what the nurse felt to be the main areas of priority (Barker 2001, 2003). Among the other reasons for this approach are:

- To respect Marion and regard her as an individual whose life experiences amount to more than information to be gathered for the purposes of documentation.
- Allowing the person to lead the assessment gives them control and responsibility, which are important in contributing to their recovery rather than the professional assuming power.
- People feel more relaxed and less anxious when permitted to provide information in their own words.
- This method allows the person to relate events as they happened for them and the person feels that they have been understood.
- The conversation provides the nurse with the opportunity to better understand Marion and her hopes and aspirations
- It provides the opportunity to begin a therapeutic relationship.

The nurse listened actively and frequently summarized what had been said to ensure that she correctly understood what Marion meant. However, the discussion may not provide all of the information the nurse needs to know, and at certain appropriate points in the conversation the nurse tactfully asked questions to prompt Marion.

Even though it was conducted as a conversation, the assessment was comprehensive, and included consideration of:

- Marion's relationships;
- family;
- housing;
- education;
- ideas for employment;
- leisure;
- spirituality;
- her relationship with her illness.

6   **Following the assessment, the nurse from the CRHT team agreed a care plan with Marion. What objectives do you think might have been identified in this plan?**

A   Due to the nature of this mental health problem, people with bipolar disorder often pose a high level of risk because of the rapid and extreme mood changes involved. However, it is important that risk assessments are not defensive exercises but instead are actively used to support people through developing meaningful risk management plans.

It was necessary for the nurse to discuss a risk management and crisis plan. The risk management plan covered a range of potential personal, social or environmental triggers, and early warning symptoms of relapse.

Risk covers a range of areas which briefly cover:

- suicide;
- harm of self and others;
- exploitation of self and others, for example, sexually or financially;
- neglect of self and dependants.

After carrying out the detailed risk assessment and developing the risk management plan, Marion was believed to present a low level of risk at the present time. However, it is necessary to continue to update risk assessments on a frequent basis as part of the care plan, as the level and nature of risk will vary greatly and sometimes rapidly for people with bipolar disorder.

The CRHT was able to monitor Marion's concordance with her medication, assess her mental state on an ongoing basis and provide psychological support based on a CBT approach. These interactions respected Marion's right to make decisions in her care and promoted her autonomy and sense of self-determination consistent with a recovery-focused approach. The recovery approach has attained a high priority within mental health services, and recognizes that empowerment is essential for people in regaining and optimizing their mental health, but this has been a difficult change to implement when professionals routinely assume a monopoly of power within the therapeutic relationship (Cleary and Dowling 2009). The recovery approach instead seeks to shift the power balance away from medical professionals, and requires therapeutic relationships to be formed on a quite different basis, with professionals eschewing power and instead recognizing the person as the expert in their care and helping them to achieve their own goals and aspirations.

Marion was given the freedom to make decisions about her care and the setting of goals. The team regularly visited her to offer support in talking about issues which were concerning her, how she was coping, whether she was taking her medication and if she was experiencing any side effects. Many of the skills needed by the nurses to promote Marion's recovery are underpinned by *The Ten Essential Shared Capabilities* (DoH 2004b) and the *Capabilities for Inclusive Practice* (DoH 2007), which promote a person-centred approach.

After involvement with the team for eight weeks, Marion felt she had more control of her mental health. Marion experienced gains in several areas, for example, her mood became more stable, and she felt she enjoyed life to a greater extent and was more optimistic and hopeful of the future. Marion was discharged back to the care of her GP with ongoing support from a **community mental health nurse** (CMHN).

REFERENCES

American Psychiatric Association (APA) (2000) *Diagnostic and Statistical Manual of Mental Disorders*, 4th edn, text version. Washington, DC: APA.

Barker, P. (2001) The Tidal Model: developing and empowering person-centred approach to recovery within psychiatric and mental health nursing, *Journal of Psychiatric and Mental Health Nursing*, 8: 233–40.

Barker, P. (2003) *Psychiatric and Mental Health Nursing: The Craft of Caring*. London: Edward Arnold Ltd.

Barker, P. (2009) *Psychiatric and Mental Health Nursing: The Craft of Caring*, 2nd edn. London: Edward Arnold Ltd.

Cleary, A. and Dowling, M. (2009) The road to recovery, *Mental Health Practice*, 12(5): 28–31.

DoH (Department of Health) (1998) *Modernizing Mental Health Services: Safe, Sound and Supportive*. London: Department of Health.

DoH (Department of Health) (1999) *National Service Framework for Mental Health: Modern Standards and Service Models*. London: DoH.

DoH (Department of Health) (2004a) *The National Service Framework for Mental Health: Five Years On*. London: DoH.

DoH (Department of Health) (2004b) *The Ten Essential Shared Capabilities: A Framework for the Whole of the Mental Health Workforce*. London: DoH.

DoH (Department of Health) (2007) *Capabilities for Inclusive Practice*. London: DoH.

Duffy, A., Alda, M., Hajek, T. and Grof, P. (2009) Early course of bipolar disorder in high-risk offspring: prospective study, *British Journal of Psychiatry*, 195: 457–8.

Fava, M. and Papakostas, G.I. (2002) *Pharmacotherapy for Depression and Treatment-Resistant Depression*. New York: World Scientific Publishing USA.

Geddes, J.R., Goodwin, G.M., Rednell, J., Azorin, J.M., Cipriani, A., Ostacher, M.I. et al. (2010) Lithium plus valproate combination therapy versus monotherapy for relapse prevention in bipolar 1 disorder (BALANCE): a randomized open-label trial, *The Lancet*, 375: 385–95.

Healy, D. (2002) *The Creation of Psychopharmacology*. Cambridge, MA: Harvard University Press.

James, R. and Gilliland, B. (2005) *Crisis Intervention Strategies*, 5th edn. New York: Thomson-Brooks.

Kessler, R.C., Berglund, P., Demler, O., Koretz, D., Rush, A.T., Waters, E.E. and Wang, P. (2003) The epidemiology of major depressive disorder: results from the national comorbidity survey replication (NCS-R), *JAMA*, 289: 2095–3105.

Morgan, S. (2000) *Clinical Risk Management- A clinical tool and practitioner manual*. London: Sainsbury Centre for Mental Health Publication.

NICE (National Institute for Health and Clinical Excellence) (2010) *The Management of Bipolar Disorder in Adults, Children and Adolescents, in Primary and Secondary Care*. London: NICE.

Norman, I. and Ryrie, I. (2009) *The Art and Science of Mental Health Nursing: A Textbook of Principles and Practice*, 2nd edn. Maidenhead: Open University Press.

Repper, J. and Perkins, R. (2003) *Social Inclusion and Recovery: A Model for Mental Health Practice.* London: Baillière Tindall.

Ryan, T. (1999) *Managing Crisis and Risk in Mental Health Nursing.* Cheltenham: Stanley Thornes Ltd.

Sachs, G.S., Printz, D.J., Kahn, D.A., Carpenter, D., et al. (2000) *Medication Treatment of Bipolar Disorder:* The Expert Consensus Guideline Series. USA

Watkins, P. (2007) *Recovery: A Guide for Mental Health Practitioners.* London: Churchill Livingstone.

World Health Organization (WHO) (1992) *ICD-10: The ICD-10 Classification of Mental and Behavioural Disorders: Clinical Descriptions and Diagnostic Guidelines.* London: Gaskell/Royal College of Psychiatrists.

Young, A.H. and Macpherson, H. (2011) Detection of bipolar disorder, *British Journal of Psychiatry,* 199: 3–4.

PART 5
Mental Health Problems in Older Adults

CASE STUDY 23
Depression in older adults
Nick Wrycraft

Ivy is 76 years old and lives alone in a bungalow she bought 18 months ago with her husband Derek. They were both looking forward to moving to a seaside town where they had enjoyed many happy family holidays together. However, a year ago, Derek had a heart attack and died.

Ivy has a small family circle with her only relatives being her daughter and sister who both live some distance away. Ivy does not see her daughter very often, as she is a single parent and has to work long hours to support her two teenage children. Ivy and her sister have never been close and rarely speak.

Concerned at not seeing Ivy recently, a neighbour contacted the police who called on her and in turn involved the mental health services. A psychiatrist visited Ivy and found the home in an untidy state and, in spite of it being mid-afternoon, Ivy appeared to have just got out of bed and appeared tired. She also seemed to have difficulty with mobility. There was very little food in the house, and Ivy seemed to have lost weight in contrast to her appearance in recent pictures in the home. Ivy was low in mood and motivation and with little hope for the future.

The psychiatrist considered discussing with Ivy that she might be admitted to an in-patient ward, however, instead felt that community-based support might be more beneficial for her situation in the longer term. With her agreement she was referred to the community mental health team and **day hospital** for a comprehensive assessment of her mental health.

1 **What might a comprehensive assessment of Ivy's mental health involve?**

A
- general mood and motivation;
- sleeping;
- eating;
- general health status;
- current medical issues and illnesses;
- past medical history, and previous illnesses;
- medication (both prescribed and non-prescribed);
- social network;
- hobbies and interests;
- hopes and aspirations for the future;
- any concerns she has over her housing or finances.

All of the above areas will be considered in a comprehensive mental health assessment. Depending on individual circumstances, some of these will be focused on to a greater extent than others.

ASSESSMENT

At the assessment at the day hospital, Ivy was unkempt, and she appeared to be very thin and pale and to move with some difficulty. Ivy had never been to a mental health centre before and appeared to be cautious and unsure of what to expect.

Ivy met with a doctor and nurse who welcomed her, introduced themselves and explained the purpose of the meeting. They then asked Ivy to explain her situation in her own words. Initially Ivy avoided eye contact, her head was lowered, her facial expression lacked animation and she spoke in a quiet, monotonous tone of voice at a slow pace. Ivy expressed doubt as to how the mental health services might be of help to her as she was a 'hopeless' case.

When speaking, Ivy often hesitated and the doctor and nurse prompted her with questions or comments to encourage her to continue speaking. At times, Ivy stopped in mid-sentence, saying she forgot what she was going to say, but after a brief pause continued. Ivy's manner seemed to be laboured and lethargic. She looked tired and said she felt as though everything was an effort.

Ivy described how following Derek's death she had found it difficult to cope, feeling a loss of purpose in life. She no longer enjoyed her previous interests and found concentrating on reading or watching television difficult; she felt a constant sense of sadness and unhappiness and was often tearful.

Although she was previously proud of and paid attention to her appearance and having a clean house, Ivy admitted that she had been 'letting things go' and no longer caring.

Ivy said that although having recently moved to the area, she had struggled to meet new people but still kept in touch with a number of friends from where she used to live with regular phone calls; this has stopped, as she said: 'they don't want to hear some moaning old woman' and that she felt she had nothing to talk about.

Ivy said that she had stopped going out of the house due to losing confidence and also as her mobility has become limited, due to osteoarthritis in her hips giving her constant pain whilst exceeding the medication which she is prescribed. Ivy has also lost interest in cooking as there is just her to cater for now and it is not worth the effort, and so when she feels hungry she eats biscuits or cold snacks but often does not feel hungry.

When asked about sleep, Ivy said that she used to sleep very well but as she has got older she sleeps much less and often only gets four or five restless hours a night and often stays in bed in the daytime, as she has nothing to get up for. However, in spite of feeling low, she has never wished she were not alive any more, and could not imagine a situation where she would feel it necessary to end her life.

In terms of previous mental health history, Ivy experienced post-natal depression following the birth of her daughter but has never experienced a mental health problem before and is not aware of any mental illness in her family.

2 **How have the doctor and nurse acted to positively engage Ivy and why is this important?**

A It is important that the person always feels empowered and that this is established as part of the relationship with healthcare professionals from the outset. Ivy was entering a new environment and unsure of what to expect. By introducing themselves, welcoming Ivy and explaining the purpose of the meeting, the doctor and nurse were demonstrating transparency, providing her with useful information and treating her with respect.

Ivy was asked to explain her story in her own words, which serves multiple purposes:

- Ivy is being listened to by the doctor and the nurse.
- As Ivy has limited social contact, she may not often receive the opportunity to explain how she feels, and this has the potential to be highly therapeutic for her.
- The doctor and nurse can appreciate how Ivy perceives her problems and what she prioritizes.

At times, Ivy stopped talking and the doctor and nurse prompted her with comments and questions. These demonstrate that they are listening, interested in what she is saying and might provide much needed reassurance, as due to her low mood, Ivy might not feel that what she has to say is of value. However, it is important that reasonable silences and gaps in the conversation are observed. Often, as in Ivy's case, people with depression can feel as though their thinking is slowed down and experience lethargy, which, if the healthcare professional speeds up the pace of conversation, can harm the development of an effective rapport. Instead it is important to work at the person's pace. It is also helpful to provide frequent summaries and to check understanding of what the person has said to ensure accuracy.

The assessment provides a good opportunity to establish a good rapport and begin working therapeutically with Ivy.

3 **What characteristics might indicate that Ivy is depressed?**

A Depression is an **affective disorder** characterized by the loss of enjoyment of life, and evident in the form of pervasive low mood, and a number of other features which are a significant alteration from the person's normal functioning. These features include behavioural, cognitive, emotional and physical factors (APA 2000; NCCMH 2011).

Applied to Ivy's case, the features of depression which she might be experiencing include behavioural features. This was apparent in Ivy's verbal and non-verbal communication, indicated as:

- subdued manner;
- low tone of voice;
- monotonous and slow rate of speech;
- avoiding eye contact;
- head in a lowered position.

More widely in the person's life, it may also be apparent in their avoiding social events or situations where they have to come into contact with others.

Cognitive features of depression are often indicated by people with depression experiencing negative and self-critical thoughts. This is evident at the beginning of the assessment, where Ivy said that she doubted whether the mental health services could help her as she was a 'hopeless' case. Ivy's experience of negative thoughts is also evident in her no longer calling her friends because 'they don't want to hear some moaning old woman'.

The types of negative thoughts people with depression experience differ, but frequently include:

- self-blame and guilt;
- doubt and loss of confidence and ruminating on problems;
- self-criticism;
- low self-esteem and worthlessness.

The person may also often experience mental lethargy and loss of motivation, which Ivy describes in terms of no longer taking a pride in her personal appearance or home, and 'letting things go'. Often in depression the person may stop activities they used to enjoy, due to no longer being able to concentrate or losing confidence, and in Ivy's case she no longer reads or watches the television or goes out.

During the assessment, Ivy often stopped mid-sentence saying that she forgot what she was going to say. Ivy also said that she feels that she has nothing to talk about and that is the reason for no longer phoning her friends. Often depression can be experienced as a slowing down of thinking, and the person may have problems finding words, or an absence of thought which is sometimes called '**poverty of thought**'. Difficulty with word finding and accessing thoughts and responding in conversation are also apparent where the person has cognitive impairment, which is a quite different mental health problem and worth investigating further.

Emotional features of depression are indicated as often people with depression can feel a sense of numbness and loss of **emotion**, for example, Ivy lacks animation and expression when speaking. However, they may also feel an overwhelming and enduring sense of powerful negative feelings, which is also the case for Ivy, as she has a constant sense of sadness and unhappiness but is also often tearful.

Physical features of depression are shown as Ivy has lost weight which is commonly a feature of depression although sometimes people gain in weight. Ivy also sleeps less (insomnia) and experiences restless sleep which leaves her feeling unrefreshed upon waking; alternatively, people with depression can also sleep excessively (hypersomnia).

Another physical aspect of depression is tiredness and lethargy, as even in the case of excessive sleeping, the person can still be tired and exhausted, due to the other features of depression which they are experiencing.

There is also a high incidence of co-morbidity of physical ill health and mental ill-health, with, on the one hand, the psychological illness of depression being evident in the form of somatic or physical symptoms where the person has illnesses and physical aches or pains which seem to be due to their mood. Alternatively, depression can be caused by the pain, discomfort and limitations to quality of life imposed by physical illness. In the case of Ivy, her osteoarthritis exerts an influence on the behavioural, cognitive and emotional features of depression.

4 **What causes depression?**

A The cause of depression is not known. However, there are a number of explanatory theories. The effectiveness of anti-depressant medication in improving the balance of chemicals in the brain and mood is often regarded as evidence that depression is a physiological issue. While this appears to be supported by the fact that people with depression often also have relatives with the same problem indicating a genetic predisposition, another interpretation of the same fact is that negative coping mechanisms are learned and also acquired behaviour.

As depression is far more prevalent among women than men, and there are a range of predisposing factors in terms of social and environmental factors including economic, educational, environmental and housing aspects, there also seems to be a sociological element involved with people's experience of depression (NCCMH 2011). Therefore, depression seems not only to be experienced in many areas of the person's functioning but to be composed of a range of factors, each of which contributes in a different but specific way.

Often depression can occur in response to stressful life events. Moving home with the unexpected bereavement of Derek in a short space of time was highly traumatic for Ivy and she experienced two life events which are recognized causes of high levels of stress (Holmes and Rahe 1967).

5   **What do you feel are the main priorities for Ivy's care plan emerging from the assessment?**

A   At the end of the assessment meeting the doctor and nurse agreed the priorities for her care with Ivy. These were:

- to address her pain from the osteoarthritis;
- to access help in improving her low mood;
- to assess her functioning at home in everyday activities.

In order to meet these goals, a number of measures were identified for Ivy's care plan, which are summarized in Table 23.1.

Ivy's CPN was her **Care Programme Approach (CPA)** coordinator, as the professional most involved with her care. The importance of the role of the care coordinator is often overlooked but they are essential for the following reasons:

- The care coordinator provides a point of contact for other professionals and the person's relatives or significant others.
- They can instigate further action when the person's needs change.
- The care coordinator ensures that communication occurs between the professionals involved in the person's care.

At her CPA meeting after 6 weeks, Ivy reported feeling improved in mood, and that she is sleeping for longer. While she has not gained in weight, she is no longer losing weight. The staff and Ivy agree that attending the day hospital has given her structure to her week and she feels this has generated an interest in the world around her. Although Ivy still often feels negative and low, overall she feels more positive about her life and that she can enjoy things and engage in the interests she used to have. She has made friendships with other people who attend the day hospital and has a good rapport with her CPN. It was agreed to plan for Ivy to attend a social services day centre in the future and attend a local lunch club on a regular basis, while Ivy plans to move to a residential home which organizes social events.

Table 23.1 Measures for Ivy's care plan

Measure	Rationale
Ivy attended an appointment with her GP who carried out a full examination, referred her to a pain specialist who changed her existing medication and provided her with additional medication for use when the pain became worse	To identify any other physical health problems which Ivy might be experiencing and to better manage the pain from her osteoarthritis and reduce the effect this has on her mood and other areas of functioning, such as sleep and nutrition
Ivy was prescribed anti-depressant medication. The effect on her mood and any possible contraindications were to be monitored by her community psychiatric nurse (CPN) and the staff at the day hospital	Anti-depressant medication is identified as being effective in the treatment of depression (NCCMH 2011)
For Ivy to attend the day hospital twice a week on Tuesdays and Thursdays and to participate in a programme of group activities including current affairs and news and group discussions	Attendance at the day hospital gave structure to Ivy's week and also offered her social inclusion (SEU 2004). Being involved with the groupwork programme encouraged Ivy to re-engage with her previous interests and performed a therapeutic function
	Guidance suggests the use of a range of psychological therapies with people experiencing depression (NCCMH 2011)
For Ivy to eat a cooked lunch and to be weighed each week while at the day hospital	Eating at the day hospital encouraged Ivy's appetite, while being weighed helped the staff to identify any further weight loss
Ivy's memory was assessed at the day hospital	Assessing Ivy's memory was useful in identifying whether her difficulties were due to struggling with thinking due to depressed mood, or cognitive impairment for which there is a different treatment pathway which is best accessed at the earliest point
A CPN visited Ivy at home initially once each week to provide support	The CPN developed a rapport with Ivy and assessed her mental state on an ongoing basis in her home environment. Ivy identified that she wanted to sleep better as her preferred goal and the CPN focused on a range of measures which she might use
An **occupational therapist (OT)** visited Ivy at home to assess her functioning	The OT can identify areas of functioning where Ivy has difficulty and make suggestions for overcoming these issues or for aids in making tasks easier

REFERENCES

APA (American Psychiatric Association) (2000) *Diagnostic and Statistical Manual of Psychiatric Disorders*, text revision. Washington, DC: APA.

Holmes, T. and Rahe, R. (1967) The Social Readjustment Rating Scale, *Journal of Psychosomatic Research*, 11: 213–18.

NCCMH (National Collaborating Centre for Mental Health) (2011) *Common Mental Health Disorders: Identification and Pathways to Care*. National Clinical Guideline Number 123. London: NICE.

NICE (National Institute for Health and Clinical Excellence) (2009) *Depression: The Treatment and Management of Depression in Adults*. London: NICE.

NMC (Nursing and Midwifery Council) (2008) *Standards of Conduct, Performance and Ethics for Nurses and Midwives*. London: NMC.

SEU (Social Exclusion Unit) (2004) *Mental Health and Social Exclusion*. London: Office of the Deputy Prime Minister.

Ruby is 68 years old and has been widowed for two years. Since losing her husband of 40 years, she has found it increasingly difficult to cope. Their son Greg lives in Australia with his wife and two children. Ruby has visited Greg in the past with her husband, but since his death she does not feel that she could make the journey.

Her GP has got to know her quite well over the last few years as she has regularly seen her for a number of complaints. Ruby explained to the GP that she felt anxious and depressed since the death of her husband and was finding it difficult to cope. Her symptoms were consistent with depression and anxiety associated with the death of her husband. Initially the GP gave Ruby a prescription of a Selective Serotonin Reuptake Inhibitor (SSRI) anti-depressant drug paroxetine 20 mg to be taken in the morning.

However, after several months, Ruby stopped taking these, stating that they did not work. Recently Ruby's visits to the GP have increased, and she has complained of increasing anxiety and sleeplessness. The GP prescribed **diazepam**, stating to her that this would only be for a short period. However, the GP now has concerns that Ruby has become dependent on diazepam, as she has attended the surgery in an agitated state several times without an appointment and been aggressive towards the reception staff demanding a prescription for more diazepam.

1   **Is Ruby an older person? At what age do people become regarded as old?**

A   According to the World Health Organization (2011), **old age** applies to people between 60–65 years. For some people this may not seem old but in Western society, this is the age when most people retire from work. However, people are increasingly working for longer, and there are proposals to increase the age of retirement for men to 66 and women to 65 with the aim of making it 66 years for both men and women by 2020 (Age UK 2011; Press Association 2011). While this could impose a physical strain on people being required to work for longer, it could also improve social inclusion and society's perceptions of older people with them being seen as still active members of the community.

Furthermore, over recent decades our life expectancy has increased with many more people living to be over 80 (BBC 2011; NHS Choices 2011) and up to 100. However, stereotypical perceptions are often applied to older people with expectations of their being prone to illness and dependence. Yet because old age applies to a longer span of years, the concept therefore embraces a wide range of diverse people. For example, a person aged 60 is generally likely to enjoy better physical and mental health than a person aged 85, yet both are regarded as elderly (Burrow 2011). As a result, an additional age banding of **very old age** has been developed to describe the increasingly large group of people who are 80 and older. Locating the threshold of this banding at 80 is significant, as this is approximately the current lifespan expectancy of adults within the UK, although women are still expected to live longer than men and there are major variations among different regions. Therefore, as people are living longer, our understanding of ageing is changing which has the potential to challenge existing stereotypical perceptions.

2   **Is it possible to become dependent upon prescription drugs?**

A   Prescription drugs can be as addictive and problematic as their illegal counterparts. There have been reports of an increase in the prescribing of anxiolytic medication, in particular tranquillizers and hypnotics to older people in both **primary** and **secondary care**. There has also been a substantial increase in the use of anxiolytic drugs worldwide, mirroring the increased use of **benzodiazepines** in the UK (INCB 2008).

Among the reasons for this are:

- Fewer older people use psychological interventions and are therefore more likely to accept medication as the only treatment which is available (White-Campbell 2011).
- An increased incidence of depression or depressive type symptoms among this client group due to life events, for example, bereavement, social isolation and economic difficulties as many older people live on a fixed limited income
- Increased contact with the health services due to physical health problems among this age group leading to greater likelihood of the detection of depressive symptoms. Physical health problems often lead to co-morbid depression.
- Healthcare professionals are more likely to perceive depressive symptoms in older people.

Benzodiazepines are part of the hypnotic and anxiolytic group of drugs. Their aim is to help alleviate anxiety, insomnia and to aid muscle relaxation. They are mainly prescribed in the short term because of their addictiveness and adverse effects (Table 24.1); however, they are beneficial in relieving acute conditions after causal factors have been established, such as bereavement or major life events in which the person is unable to cope (BNF 2011).

From a psychological perspective, they are normally prescribed for a short period of between 4–6 weeks for generalized anxiety, insomnia, phobias and obsessive compulsive disorders. However, they are also prescribed for physical problems such as organic disorders (such as liver failure) and feelings of inner restlessness leading the person to become excessively active (**akathisia**) (Levi 2007).

Ruby's GP decided to make a home visit to discuss why she is coming to the surgery demanding additional diazepam. During this visit Ruby confides that she has been using more of her prescription than normal. This is because she is not sleeping and is becoming increasingly anxious and depressed. She believes that the diazepam helps her to keep calm and helps her sleep. Her current prescription is diazepam 2 mg three times daily. However, she says that she was unable to sleep and took double the dose one night. Ruby then felt a need to increase again and has been taking 10 mg daily and now has insufficient medication to last until the next prescription. She states that she is now less anxious and can sleep at night. Ruby is adamant that the GP has not been giving her the proper dose of diazepam and wants her prescription increased.

Table 24.1 Benzodiazepines: hypnotics and anxiolytics

Drug	Indication	Adverse (side) effects
Hypnotics Nitrazepam Flurazepam Loprazolam Lormetazepam Temazepam	Usually given for insomnia	Drowsiness, light-headedness (the next day), confusion and ataxia (especially in the older person), overdose and dependency
Anxiolytics Diazepam Alprazolam (Chlordiazepoxide hydrochloride) Lorazepam Oxazepam	Usually given for anxiety	As above, plus headache, hypotension, vertigo, tremor, visual and gastric disturbances Urinary retention

Note: See BNF (2011) for a full explanation of benzodiazepines.

The GP was concerned about Ruby self-medicating, as especially among older people there is an increased risk of overdose with benzodiazepines due to tolerance decreasing with age (Rassool 2011). Diazepam can also quickly become addictive and so may cause more problems than it was originally prescribed to solve (Pycroft 2010).

Diazepam should not be:

* prescribed for more than four weeks.

Diazepam should be prescribed (Levi 2007):

* within therapeutic dose ranges beginning 2 mg three times daily (6 mg);
* with a maximum of 10 mg three times daily (30 mg).

There is also the potential for overdose if the drug is taken in larger doses or with a combination of other drugs such as alcohol.

3 **What should the GP do to promote Ruby's physical and mental health?**

A
* The GP immediately arranged for a full physical health check, to identify any ill effects from Ruby taking in excess of the prescribed dosage of diazepam.
* The GP involved services which can offer Ruby more in-depth support and monitoring. Among the options are:
  * the **community mental health team (CMHT)**;
  * the Improving Access to Psychological Therapies (IAPT) team.

COMMUNITY MENTAL HEALTH TEAM (CMHT)

Community mental health teams (CMHTs) are provided by specialist secondary mental health services, and are part of a network of community-based mental health services. These include:

- **Assertive outreach** providing ongoing support for people with severe and enduring **long-term mental health problems**;
- Child and Adolescent Mental Health Services (CAMHS) for children with mental health problems;
- **Criminal Justice and Court diversion**, liaising with the Courts to provide mental health assessments and reports for people in the Criminal Justice system;
- Crisis Resolution and Home Treatment (CRHT) teams to provide brief and time-limited support and intervention for people experiencing crisis in the community;
- **Early Intervention in Psychosis (EiP)** to facilitate rapid access to services for younger adults experiencing acute mental health problems;
- **Substance misuse teams** to support people with drug and alcohol issues;
- **Youth Offending Teams (YoTs)** work with younger people who have come into contact with the Criminal Justice system.

However, unlike many of the teams listed above who work with a very specific client group, CMHTs work with a range of people with different mental health problems. Often they receive referrals from GPs to provide additional support for people experiencing mental health problems.

The CMHT comprises a range of staff from different disciplines who offer a full range of skills with which to help the service user, including:

- doctors trained in mental health;
- mental health nurses;
- occupational therapists (OTs);
- psychologists;
- social workers;
- Support Time and Recovery (STR) workers.

The aim of the team is:

- to offer a comprehensive psychological assessment;
- to provide a personalized and collaborative plan of care, including ongoing support and therapeutic interventions;
- to promote recovery.

The care of all people with whom the CMHT are involved is regularly reviewed in accordance with the Care Programme Approach (CPA) which aims to provide comprehensive individualized care flexible to individual needs.

The Improving Access to Psychological Therapies (IAPT) programme is a Department of Health initiative, introduced in 2005 to improve access to psychological therapies within primary care. This followed on from the government's White Paper, *Our Health, Our Care, Our Say* (DoH 2006). IAPT services are available as low intensity or high intensity. Low intensity services work with common mental health problems such as Ruby is experiencing in depression and anxiety, while the high intensity service work with people with severe and enduring conditions such as schizophrenia.

Low intensity IAPT services do the following:

* offer a limited number of sessions;
* provide brief interventions including behavioural activation, cognitive restructuring, graded exposure, medication management, problem solving and sleep hygiene;
* have the potential to be delivered flexibly in terms of face-to-face or by telephone.

Initially IAPT was developed for people of working age; however, since it has proven so successful, it has been extended to all age groups (NHS 2011). IAPT proceeds on a five-step approach to treatment which ensures that people receive the appropriate level of treatment based on the notion that the least interventionist option is preferred (DoH 2007).

Ruby might be referred to either the CMHT or IAPT as the resources of both ensure a multi-disciplinary approach to care and practice, in accordance with the guidelines for the treatment of depression and anxiety (NCCMH 2011). However, due to the complex nature of Ruby's problem, the GP decided to involve the CMHT, as they could offer more comprehensive support and monitor her detoxification if needed.

Ruby agreed to meet the community mental health nurse (CMHN). The GP also attended the assessment. It became clear that Ruby is still grieving for her husband and struggling to cope with feeling lonely and the 'emptiness' of her days, which has made her increasingly anxious and she feels as though she is in constant turmoil. Ruby was reluctant to take the paroxetine which the GP prescribed through fear of becoming addicted, and the stigma associated with being depressed. Ruby also did not want her son to think that she could not cope. However, when Ruby was prescribed the diazepam, she felt much calmer, and for the first time in some months was able to sleep well at night. Because of the positive effect it had, Ruby did not understand why the GP could not keep prescribing her the diazepam as it was really working.

4 **What treatment is required to effectively address the issue of benzodiazepine dependence and anxiety and depression with someone of Ruby's age?**

A The strategy for treating someone with benzodiazepine dependence is for a period of stabilization and gradual reduction in the dose over a set time (Oude Voshaar et al. 2006). However, this can be a frightening experience especially for an older adult such as Ruby, as she may feel unable to cope with the prospect of not being able to rely on medication if the anxiety re-occurs.

Rebound symptoms can occur when withdrawing from benzodiazepines but this is usually the case in acute dependence. Physical symptoms may not be as obvious in mild to moderate dependency; however, some may still occur, for example, insomnia, sweating, anxiety and restlessness. There may also be longer-lasting psychological effects (Levi 2007; Oude Voshaar et al. 2006).

Psychological intervention is essential in the treatment of anxiety and depressive disorders, and there is substantial evidence to support the combined use of psychological therapies with medication (NCCMH 2011; NICE 2009). Engagement is an essential part of the process of assessment and intervention. However, this process will be impeded if healthcare professionals take the view that they are dealing with a person who is unable to take responsibility and fully participate in the process simply because they are an older adult (Table 24.2).

Table 24.2 Engagement

Barriers to engagement (older person)	Helpful engagement (professional)
Physical health problems	Positive staff attitudes to the older person
Stigma of mental health/drug or alcohol dependence	Social inclusion
Lack of trust	Supportive services
Fear of the unknown	Services to suit needs
Social isolation	Befriending service
Low self-esteem/feeling of worthlessness	Spiritual needs acknowledged and met
Financial insecurity	
Lack of family support	

There are less specialized resources in relation to the screening and treatment for the older person with anxiety/depression and substance misuse problems. Some evidence supports the use of psychotherapeutic interventions in older adults with mild depression. However, fewer older people than younger adults use psychological interventions, and are therefore more likely to accept medication as the only treatment which is available (White-Campbell 2011; Wilson et al. 2009). This could be due to ageism on the part of service providers. However, due to our tendency to experience physical health problems as we grow older, services for this age group often emphasize the provision of services for the physical needs of older people. While this might demonstrate the rationing of scarce resources, it ought not to be the case that the mental health of older adults is not provided for, especially as the population is now living for much longer and the needs of people like Ruby will inevitably increase.

Ruby fully engaged with the CMHN, and is responding well to treatment. She acknowledged, after explanation and guidance, that she needed to withdraw from diazepam and recommence the anti-depressant paroxetine. This transition was fairly straightforward as she had mild physical symptoms of addiction with a mainly psychological dependence. More importantly, Ruby was given time and support to discuss her feelings. She agreed to see a grief counsellor, which she finds immensely helpful and supportive. With support from the CMHN, she made the decision to tell her son of her depression and isolation and he is making a trip to see her with the grandchildren. Ruby still feels she has a long way to go, especially in relation to her social isolation and self-esteem, and this is something which she is now aware of and working on with the nurse. Ruby now realizes that the factors that were making her feel ill were not physical but psychological.

CONCLUSION

This case study considers the experience of Ruby who is an older adult misusing prescribed medication. Both older people and those who misuse substances are regarded within narrow stereotypical confines. Often due to no longer being actively involved with work, older people experience social exclusion and isolation within society. In reflecting on this case, it is helpful to consider how we define both old age and substance misuse and how these labels can impede effective engagement. The case study also highlights areas for development such as how services need to be flexible in order to provide effective psychological treatments for the increasing numbers of older people who will require this support in the future.

REFERENCES

Age UK (2011) http://www.ageuk.org.uk/latest-news/archive/forced-retirement-to-be-scrapped/ (accessed 25 October 2011).

BBC (2011) Life expectancy rises again, ONS says. Available at: http://www.bbc.co.uk/news/business-15372869?t=1320428766 (accessed 6 November 2011).

British Medical Association (2011) Royal Pharmaceutical Society, *British National Formulary,* p. 207. London: BMJ and Pharmaceutical Press. Available at: http://www.bnf.org/bnf/index.htm (accessed 25 October 2011).

Burrow, S. (2011) Helping older people with mental health problems, in S. Pryjmachuk (ed.) *Mental Health Nursing: An Evidence Based Introduction.* London: Sage.

DoH (Department of Health) (2007) *Improving Access to Psychological Therapies, Commissioning a Brighter Future.* Available at: http://www.mhchoice.csip.org.uk/psychological-therapies/-iapt-commissionerled-pathfinder-sites/resources.html (accessed 25 October 2011).

DoH (Department of Health) (2006) *Our Health, Our Care, Our Say: A New Direction for Community Services.* Available at: http://webarchive.nationalarchives.gov.uk/+/www.dh.gov.uk/en/Publicationsandstatistics/Publications/PublicationsPolicyAndGuidance/DH_4127453 (accessed 26 October 2011).

INCB (International Narcotics Control Board) (2008) *Report for the International Narcotics Control Board for 2008.* New York: United Nations.

Levi, M.I. (2007) *Basic Notes in Psychopharmacology,* 4th edn. Oxford: Radcliffe Publishing.

NHS (National Health Service) (2011) *Improving Access to Psychological Therapies.* Available at http://www.iapt.nhs.uk/about-iapt/about-us/ (accessed 25 October 2011).

NCCMH (National Collaborating Centre for Mental Health) (2011) National Clinical Guideline Number 123, *Common Mental Health Disorders: Identification and Pathways to Care.* London: NICE.

NHS Choices (2011) UK life expectancy still rising. Available at: http://www.nhs.uk/news/2011/03March/Pages/uk-life-expectancy-still-rising.aspx (accessed 6 November 2011).

NICE (National Institute for Health and Clinical Excellence) (2009) *Depression: The Treatment and Management of Depression in Adults.* Clinical Guideline 90. Available at: http://guidance.nice.org.uk/nicemedia/live/12329/45888/45888.pdf (accessed 25 October 2011).

Oude Voshaar, R.C., Gorgels, W.J.M.J., Mol, J.J., Van Balkon, A.J.L.M., Van De Lisdonk, E.H., Breteler, M.H.M., Van Den Hoogen, H.J.M., Zitman, F.G. (2006) Tapering off long-term benzodiazepine use with or without group cognitive-behavioural therapy: three-condition randomised controlled trial, *British Journal of Psychiatry,* 188: 188–189. Available at: http://bjp.rcpsych.org/content/188/2/188.full (accessed 10 May 2012).

Press Association (2011) Forced retirement to be scrapped, in Age UK. Available at: http://www.ageuk.org.uk/latest-news/archive/forced-retirement-to-be-scrapped/ (accessed 25 October 2011).

Pycroft, A. (2010) *Understanding and Working with Substance Misusers.* London: Sage.

Rassool, G. H. (2011) *Understanding Addiction Behaviours: Theoretical and Clinical Practice in Health and Social Care.* Basingstoke: Palgrave Macmillan.

White-Campbell, M. (2011) The older adult, in D.B. Cooper (ed.) *Practice in Mental Health: Substance Use.* Oxford: Radcliffe Publishing.

Wilson, K., Mottram, P.G. and Vassilas, C. (2009) Psychotherapeutic treatments for older depressed people, *Cochrane Database for Systematic Reviews,* issue 1. Available at: http://www2.cochrane.org/reviews/en/ab004853.html (accessed 25 October 2011).

World Health Organization (2012) *Definition of an Older or Elderly Person,* Health Statistics and Health Information Systems. Available at: http://www.who.int/healthinfo/survey/ageingdefnolder/en/index.html (accessed 28 April 2012).

FURTHER READING

Neilson, S. and Lee, N. (2011) Prescription drugs and mental health, in D.B. Cooper (ed.) *Practice in Mental Health: Substance Use.* Oxford: Radcliffe Publishing.

Mrs Jean Jones is 82 years old and was recently diagnosed as having Alzheimer's disease (AD) by the memory assessment team. Her husband, George, died four years ago following a major stroke and Jean now lives alone in a terraced house in a small, rural community. She moved there more than twenty years after retiring, following a successful career as a primary school teacher, and being a headmistress for more than ten years.

For some years Jean played an active role in the local village community, including parish council work and managing the local post office. Jean has two daughters, Clare, aged 48, and Jill, aged 46, who live about 200 miles away in a large town. Jean's daughters are married with teenage children and visit her once a month. Although neighbours and friends support Jean, they have become increasingly concerned that her memory is worsening, and have had to help her return home on a number of occasions after she was found wandering and lost in local streets, saying that she was looking for the school children to start their maths lesson.

A community psychiatric nurse (CPN) is visiting Mrs Jones for the first time. Jean welcomes the CPN to her house but states that she does not understand why they are calling, and has no recollection of being assessed at the memory clinic or of being found wandering in the street. Jean says that she is coping well and kept very busy with her parish council work.

1 **What are the early signs and symptoms of Alzheimer's disease (AD), and how are Jean's comments characteristic of this?**

A In the early stages of AD, individuals start to experience difficulties with their short-term memory and this can cause episodes of confusion. People might be aware of these changes and so may cover up or '**confabulate**' explanations for these lapses to preserve their self-esteem. Conversely people might really believe that they have recently undertaken activities that in fact they ceased to do many years ago. It is also quite common for people to believe they are living in a house from an earlier life stage and so go for walks in 'their local neighbourhood' only to become lost and disoriented. Emotional outbursts and occasional aggressive behaviour can result from being 'thwarted' in their quest to seek out old friends or their children who are now adults. Therefore Jean's behaviour and conversation can be seen to be characteristic of early AD.

Rather than using a series of assessment questions, mental health workers can pick up clues, contradictions and a lack of consistency from Jean by simply spending time with her and conducting a conversation. This is a far more sensitive and person-centred way of conducting an assessment. For example, Jean may repeat certain points and it may become clear there are gaps in her recall of events.

Research has provided valuable insights into the emotional impact of memory loss, the reduced self-esteem and reactions to diagnosis. Gillies (2000) documented the 'humiliating effects of unreliable memory', and the coping mechanisms employed. Similarly, Phinney (2008) asked 'What is it like to experience dementia?' and documented the loss of social contacts, confidence, self-esteem, dignity and respect.

2   **Alzheimer's disease is a type of dementia. How many different types of dementia are there and how is dementia defined?**

A   Dementia is an umbrella term that incorporates AD, **vascular dementia, Lewy body dementia**, mixed dementia and other rarer forms. People who have a **minor cognitive impairment** may also have an increased risk of progressing to AD.

   The proportions of people with different forms of dementia are summarized in Table 25.1, with AD the most common.

Table 25.1 Proportion of people with different forms of dementia

Dementia type	(%)
Alzheimer's disease	62
Vascular dementia	17
Mixed dementia	10
Dementia with Lewy bodies	4
Fronto-temporal dementia (including Pick's disease)	2
Parkinson's dementia	2
Other dementias (including Korsakoff's syndrome, HIV and AIDS-related dementia and Creutzfeldt-Jakob disease)	3

Source: Alzheimer's Society *Dementia UK* (2007)

Traditionally, dementia has been defined as a physical disease with a focus on **neuropathology** and the associated decline in psychological and physical functioning:

> Dementia is a degenerative brain syndrome characterised by a progressive decline in memory, thinking, comprehension, calculation, language, learning capacity and judgment sufficient to impair personal activities of daily living.
>
> (WHO 2001)

> Dementia describes a group of symptoms associated with a progressive decline of brain functions, such as memory, understanding, judgement, language and thinking. People with dementia are at an increased risk of physical health problems.
>
> (Dementia Action Alliance 2010)

Alzheimer's disease was first described by the German neurologist Alois Alzheimer in 1906, and is a physical brain disease whereby **amyloid plaques** and **neurofibrillary tangles** develop on the cerebral cortex and this causes the loss (death) of brain cells (neurons). There is also a shortage of important brain chemicals, such as acetylcholine, which are involved with the transmission of messages in the brain. Over time, more parts of the brain are damaged and so symptoms become more severe (Alzheimer's Society 2010a).

3 **How many people in the UK are currently diagnosed with dementia and by how much is this projected to increase?**

A In 2007, the following estimates of dementia per country within the UK were produced (Table 25.2).

Table 25.2 Dementia per country within the UK

Country	No. of dementia sufferers
England	574,717
Scotland	56,106
Northern Ireland	15,850
Wales	36,924
Total	683,597

Based on the figures in Table 25.2, the UK prevalence rates for dementia within the age ranges are:

40–64 years:	1 in 1400 people
65–69 years:	1 in 100
70–79 years:	1 in 25
80+ years:	1 in 6

(Alzheimer's Society 2007)

Recent reports now estimate there to be 821,884 people in the UK with dementia, of which females make up 66 per cent (Dementia Action Alliance 2010). Correspondingly, Bamford (2010) states that one person in 20 of those aged over 65 years has dementia. This is 15 per cent higher than previously estimated.

It is projected that by 2021 there will be about 940,000 people with dementia in the UK, and this is expected to rise to over 1.7 million by 2051 as the population ages, by which time 1 in 3 people over the age of 65 will have a form of dementia (Alzheimer's Society 2007; Bamford 2010).

Worldwide estimates of dementia indicate that there are nearly 25 million people with dementia, with an estimated 4.6 million new cases each year. In Europe a new case of dementia arises every 24 seconds. In France, there are 850,000 people with dementia, in Germany, 1.2 million (the highest in Europe), in Portugal, 140,000 and in Malta 4,000. The number of cases depends on the population size and how this population ages (Bamford 2010).

4 **What might cause Alzheimer's disease?**

A There seem to be a number of lifestyle factors related to AD. In 2010, the Alzheimer's Society (AS) research group convened an expert panel to review the available evidence and suggested that lifestyle factors, such as a healthy diet, high levels of physical and mental activity and social interaction can help prevent dementia. Excessive smoking and hypertension are established risk factors. Better treatment of medical problems such as high blood pressure and high cholesterol can further reduce risk.

No one single factor has been identified as causing A D so far, but is likely to be a combination of factors including age, genetic inheritance, environmental factors, diet and general health (Alzheimer's Research Trust 2010).

5   **Jean had been diagnosed with Alzheimer's disease by the memory assessment team; what services do these teams provide?**

A   The memory service receives referrals from G Ps and aims to provide prompt access to an assessment of the memory of people with symptoms of dementia. Under the National Dementia Strategy, mental health Trusts are required to provide these services locally which are delivered by a team of specialist mental health professionals.

A range of psychological (and physical) assessment methods and tools are used including the Mini-Mental State Examination (M M S E) which tests memory, knowledge and the ability to perform simple calculations. Where appropriate, assessment is followed by a diagnosis and the accessing of ongoing support, therapy and treatment if necessary (usually an **anti-cholinesterase** drug such as aricept). Following the assessment and diagnosis, a C P N has been asked to visit Jean and discuss with her, agree and then organize a care package to meet her needs.

Other diagnostic tests may include physical tests such as a review of Jean's past medical history, blood tests, a neurological exam (referral to a neurologist for testing of nervous system, co-ordination, speech, eye movement and reflexes) and brain imaging, for example, computerized tomography (C T) and magnetic resonance imaging (M R I).

From the community mental health nurse's initial assessment of Jean it becomes clear that she will require further support due to her short-term memory problems, and is also vulnerable because she lives alone. Recent research and current policy require planning care and interventions that are based on 'person-centred dementia care'.

6   **What does person-centred dementia care mean? Also what interventions would be suitable for Jean?**

A   The contemporary principles of caring for someone with dementia have been greatly influenced by the work of Kitwood (1997). Within a person-centred framework, care is based on the assumption that all humans have five fundamental psychological needs. These are:

- comfort;
- attachment;
- inclusion;
- occupation;
- identity.

Based on this assumption Kitwood studied how personhood concepts of biography and personality influence how the person experiences dementia. He also sought to understand how 'good' dementia care could be implemented through the adoption of positive person work and dementia care mapping (Kitwood 1997). This approach has helped to initiate a major shift in the focus of dementia care, to a 'person-centred approach'.

Similarly, Stokes (2008) sought to discover the meaning of 'problem' behaviours, and advocated that these should not be regarded as part of the dementia. Stokes instead suggests that while the reason for behaviour might be located in the formative years, it is important to highlight that the personality is not lost to the dementia. For example, Jean's wandering and appearing to believe she is looking for her school class is clearly a mistaken belief which places her at potential risk and so could be regarded as a problem. However, it can be explained and understood not as part of her dementia but as her personal response to her failing memory.

The NICE dementia care pathway offers excellent guidance for mental health professionals in providing person-centred care for people with dementia. In accordance with this pathway, a number of interventions need to be considered when supporting Jean at home. Table 25.3 shows the interventions to help Jean remain independent.

Table 25.3 Interventions to help Jean

Intervention	*Rationale*
Weekly home support visits by the CPN that will include monitoring of drug treatment for her dementia and assessing her physical health and nutritional needs. Jean will also require emotional support and the compilation of a personal biography	Regular home visits will be needed because this will allow continuous assessment of Jean's memory difficulties and cognitive ability. This will also allow the assessment of her self-care capabilities. The monitoring of pharmacological interventions is important to ensure concordance, access early treatment for any side effects, and to be able to ascertain the effectiveness of treatment. Jean may become distressed and depressed as a result of her dementia. The compilation of a personal biography promotes individualized care
Attendance at a **well-being centre** to include **cognitive stimulation therapy**	This will help alleviate Jean's loneliness and isolation but importantly help her retain her short-term memory for as long as possible
Attendance at a well-being centre to include physical activities	Physical activity and physical health can be important factors in slowing the psychological decline of dementia
Attendance at a well-being centre to include activities of daily living (ADL), advice and skill training from an occupational therapist	This type of skills assessment and training can be important to enable Jean to cope and be supported at home for as long as possible
Organize support from local community and clubs	Jean's neighbours and the local community have played an important role in supporting her to date and may be willing to keep a 'watching eye' out for her. Many villages have voluntary clubs and centres that play a vital role in local community life
Family involvement	It is important that her daughters and family are fully consulted and involved in Jean's care plan. There will be some difficult decisions to take in the future, e.g. financial planning, so it is vital they are involved and understand the nature of AD
Assistive technology and **telecare**	Will increase Jean's safety and support at home
Memory aids	It is possible to work with Jean to provide a number of cues and prompts around the home to enable her to maintain her routine and safety at home
Dementia café attendance	If a café is available locally, this can provide an invaluable support to Jean and her family

According to the AS fact sheet 526 (Alzheimer's Society 2010b), there are four common areas where difficulty in short-term memory is experienced: (1) remembering recent events; (2) receiving new information; (3) remembering names; and (4) separating reality from fiction as the person finds it increasingly difficult to understand events which are occurring due to memory problems. According to this fact sheet, the ways to help Jean cope with her memory difficulties include:

- using reminiscence to promote recall of positive emotions and events;
- keeping information simple with stepped activities;
- using tactful reminders to help her to recognize people;
- sensitively correcting inaccurate recall;
- helping her to avoid unnecessary stress and keep to a regular routine.

There are other therapies that might also be used to help Jean:

- Reality orientation is concerned with taking regular opportunities to sensitively orientate people with dementia in terms of the time, date, season, etc.
- Reminiscence therapy is concerned with stimulating the pleasurable recall of past memories or events by using music, video, photographs and images.
- Validation therapy is concerned with attempting to enter the inner emotional and personal world of the individual with dementia and involves seeking to develop an awareness of their feelings and the underlying meaning of their verbal communication.

The NICE dementia care pathway has been used to guide the interventions for Jean's care. This was developed to complement and support the implementation of the National Dementia Strategy.

7 **What are the main objectives of the National Dementia Strategy?**

A The National Dementia Strategy was published in February 2009 and updated in September 2010 and remains the key document in terms of the strategies that will guide dementia care in the coming three to five years. With local accountability and delivery being the main focus, there are now 18 objectives, of which the following have priority:

- good quality early diagnosis and intervention for all;
- improved community personal support services;
- a focus on carers;
- improved quality of care for people with dementia in general hospitals;
- living well with dementia in care homes;
- a joint commissioning strategy for dementia;
- a capable and effective workforce;
- reduced use of antipsychotic medication.

In addition to the National Strategy, the National Dementia Declaration, launched in October 2010, outlines seven outcomes that people with dementia and their carers say they would like to see: personal choice; support to live their life; living in an enabling environment; services designed for personal needs; knowledge to get what they need; a sense of belonging; and knowledge of research that improves quality of life. Similarly, the document, *Quality Outcomes for People with Dementia: Building on the Work of the National Dementia Strategy*, released in September 2010, identifies outcomes desired by people with dementia and their carers to be achieved by 2014, including early diagnosis, informed decision-making, the best treatment and support, family support, being treated with dignity and respect, enabling self-help, feeling part of a community, enjoying life, respect for end-of-life wishes and a good death.

8 **What role might the Alzheimer's Society (AS) play in supporting Jean?**

A The AS is a registered charity which aims to improve the quality of life for people who have dementia and their carers. Their activities include funding research, developing awareness campaigns and providing training. In terms of support to Jean, the AS provide local services including day and home care, outreach workers, befriending schemes, support groups, carer support and a point of contact and information by telephone, or on-line services.

9 **After some months of supporting Jean at home, her memory seems to be worsening and she is neglecting her personal hygiene and losing weight. What changes to her care package are necessary to meet her new needs?**

A The way that a person experiences AD will depend on many factors, including their physical characteristics, their emotional coping abilities and the support available. As can be seen from Jean's case, in the early stages there were relatively minor changes in her abilities, memory and behaviour but as the illness progressed, the changes became more apparent and she required greater support to meet her needs (Table 25.4). As Jean's memory worsens, she may be unable to recognize close relatives and friends or even her own 'older' self. This may affect her confidence and self-care abilities and so she will become increasingly dependent. In

Table 25.4 Review of interventions as Jean's memory worsens

Intervention	Rationale
Medical assessment and examination	To ensure Jean's weight loss and psychological decline are not due to other physical causes
Case review of Jean's care by the multi-disciplinary team led by her care co-ordinator	It is important to recognize and respond to any deterioration in Jean's physical and psychological well-being and to ensure that all of the skills of the professional team are fully utilized in her care
Continue emotional support and ongoing psychological interventions	Evidence-based psychological interventions are important at every stage of dementia to ensure care is person-centred
Consider increased day care at the well-being centre	This might enable Jean to remain at home for longer
Consider increased support at home by the intensive support and social care teams	Ensure her physical, social, emotional and ADL needs continue to be met

(Continued overleaf)

Table 25.4 Continued

Intervention	Rationale
Involvement and advice from specialist workers such as **Admiral nurses**	There has been considerable investment in specialist dementia care workers who will be able to suggest a range of support mechanisms for Jean
Assessment within an in-patient unit for older adults with a view to placement in a specialist residential home or shared care housing facility	It will become necessary to consider such an assessment in collaboration with Jean's daughters
	There are now a number of high quality homes specializing in the care of people with dementia

the later stages she will require even greater support and will eventually become reliant on others to meet her needs (AS 2010c). The importance of planning for palliative or end-of-life care from diagnosis is highlighted in the National Dementia Strategy and this should be focused on personal choice and high quality care that enables people with dementia like Jean to plan their end-of-life care and die with dignity (NICE 2010).

REFERENCES

Alzheimer's Disease International (2010) *World Alzheimer Report 2010: The Global Economic Impact of Dementia*. Cambridge: Alzheimer's Disease International.

Alzheimer's Research Trust (2010) *Dementia 2010: The Prevalence, Economic Cost and Research Funding of Dementia Compared with Other Diseases*. London: Alzheimer's Research Trust.

Alzheimer's Society (AS) (2007) *Dementia UK: A Report to the Alzheimer's Society on the Prevalence and Economic Cost of Dementia in the UK by King's College, London and the London School of Economics*. London: Alzheimer's Society.

Alzheimer's Society (AS) (2010a) *What Is Alzheimer's Disease?* Fact sheet number 401. London: Alzheimer's Society.

Alzheimer's Society (AS) (2010b) *Coping with Memory Loss*. Fact sheet number 526. London: Alzheimer's Society.

Alzheimer's Society (AS) (2010c) *The Later Stages of Dementia*. Fact sheet number 417. London: Alzheimer's Society.

Alzheimer's Society (AS) (2010d) *What Is Dementia?* Fact sheet number 400. London: Alzheimer's Society.

Alzheimer's Society (AS) (2010e) *Assistive Technology: Devices to Help with Everyday Living*. Fact sheet number 437. London: Alzheimer's Society.

Alzheimer's Society (AS) (2010f) *Mild Cognitive Impairment*. Fact sheet number 470. London: Alzheimer's Society.

Bamford, S. (2010) Tackling dementia across the Channel, *Community Care*, 22 April.

Dementia Action Alliance (2010) *Delivering the National Dementia Declaration for England: Action Plans 2010–2014*. London: Dementia Action Alliance.

Department of Health (2009) *Living Well with Dementia: A National Dementia Strategy*. London: The Stationery Office.

Department of Health (2010) *Quality Outcomes for People with Dementia: Building on the Work of the National Dementia Strategy*. London: The Stationery Office.

Gillies, B.A. (2000) A memory like clockwork: accounts of living through dementia, *Aging & Mental Health*, 4(4): 366–74.

Kitwood, T. (1997) *Dementia Reconsidered: The Person Comes First*. Buckingham: Open University Press.

NICE (National Institute for Health and Clinical Excellence) (2010) *Dementia Quality Standard*. London: NICE.

Phinney, A. (2008) Toward understanding subjective experiences of dementia, in M. Downes and B. Bowers (eds) *Excellence in Dementia Care*. Maidenhead: McGraw-Hill.

Stokes, G. (2008) *And Still the Music Plays*. London: Hawker.

WHO (World Health Organization) (2001) *When Old Age Becomes a Disease*. WHO: Mumbai.

WEB RESOURCES

Alzheimer's Society
http://www.alzheimers.org.uk/

Care programme approach
http://www.dh.gov.uk/en/Publicationsandstatistics/Publications/PublicationsPolicyAndGuidance/DH_083647

Carers UK web page
http://www.carersuk.org/

Department of Health carers page
http://www.dh.gov.uk/en/SocialCare/Carers/index.htm

Memory assessment guidance
http://www.nice.org.uk/usingguidance/commissioningguides/memoryassessmentservice/memoryassessmenthome.jsp

National Dementia Strategy
http://www.dh.gov.uk/en/SocialCare/NationalDementiaStrategy/index.htm

National Institute for Health and Clinical Excellence Dementia Care Guidance
http://guidance.nice.org.uk/CG42

National Institute for Health and Clinical Excellence Dementia Care Pathway
http://pathways.nice.org.uk/pathways/dementia

John Chan is 72 years old and the main carer for his 70-year-old wife, Daphne. The couple live in a large city in a comfortable, well-maintained detached house. Their two sons and three daughters all live close by and so Mr and Mrs Chan are reasonably well supported by their extended family and teenage grandchildren. The Chinese couple moved to England from Hong Kong in the 1970s and both enjoyed relatively long careers with John working in the finance sector and Daphne in accountancy.

Over the past thirty years Daphne has had to take periods of sick leave from her work because she became very anxious and concerned that she was not sufficiently thorough in her accountancy work, and so spent many additional hours repeatedly checking figures and statistics. Eventually she was diagnosed with obsessive compulsive disorder (OCD) and, as a result, Mrs Chan was admitted to an in-patient mental health unit on a number of occasions.

Daphne has also received cognitive behavioural therapy (CBT), and been prescribed anxiolytic drugs. At the age of 56, Daphne had to take early retirement, and has recently become increasingly depressed and agitated. She is currently being supported at home by a community mental health nurse, but during their most recent visit her husband stated that he is finding it increasingly difficult to cope due to Daphne's agitation and worsening low mood. John also mentions that he is starting to experience muscle and joint pain, indigestion and palpitations.

1 **Are there many situations like John and Daphne's with one person caring for the other with a mental health problem?**

A As Daphne's carer, John is one of the 1.5 million UK carers providing practical and emotional support to people affected by mental health difficulties (DoH 2002). It is anticipated this number will increase once the **National Census** data collected in 2011 is released.

Carers may be a husband, wife, partner, family member or friend (Rethink 2006). Caring for someone with mental health needs such as Daphne is a considerable undertaking that can cause social disruption and even financial difficulties (Weinberg and Huxley 2000). Despite recent improvements in community mental health care, a heavy burden continues to be placed on **informal carers** with their lives often becoming chaotic as a result of the responsibilities which this entails. Carers frequently have to completely restructure their lives to meet the demands of caring and such changes can often detrimentally affect their physical and emotional health (DoH 2002). The effect of caring can be so great that some mental health carers feel that they are 'invisible and silent partners' in care and under-valued by the care services (Sin et al. 2005).

2 **Which factors would you consider to be of particular importance in your assessment of Mr Chan's personal situation?**

A The impact of caring for Mrs Chan can be seen to correlate with the concept of objective and subjective carer burden as described by Morris (1991). Objective burden refers to the practical impact, the physical health effects and the daily routine changes. Subjective burden relates to the carers' emotional reaction and perception of strain, including morale, anxiety, depression and loss of social contacts. On assessing John using this framework, the following needs can be identified (Table 26.1).

3 **How might cultural factors influence the type of support that John might accept?**

A A person's cultural background will affect their interpretation of illness, and the impact of culture is an important determinant of whether, or at what point, an individual will ask for **medical intervention** (Cheng 2001). Such a cultural phenomenon becomes even more influential when seeking help for mental illness (Kung and Lu 2008). In Chinese culture, a somatic

Table 26.1 Objective and subjective burdens of caring

Objective burden	Rationale	Subjective burden	Rationale
Physical effects of anxiety experienced as a result of John's caring role	Anxiety, depression and stress are common manifestations of the caring role	Frustration at being unable to discuss his feelings about his caring situation	Cultural and gender issues might make it difficult for John to express his feelings
The personal impact of routine change disrupted sleep and a lack of physical exercise	The consequence of caring for someone with a mental illness can include sleep loss and other physical effects Anxiety manifesting as the somatic complaints he mentions such as muscle and joint pain and palpitations Anxiety might be the result of a loss of his work role or reluctance to seek help	Potential loss of friends and work colleagues	Informal carers often mention the loss of social networks Frequently this is because friends become unsure how to respond Where stress is prolonged, physical complaints are common Resentment can result from the loss of work role following retirement or having to restructure one's life around caring. The impact of this is often determined by the quality of the relationship

or physical complaint is perceived as a more legitimate reason than a psychological one for seeking help (Barsky 1992). This is because a person's physical condition is central to their daily lives and conversely feelings of anxiety and depression are likely to be less prioritized (Kung and Lu 2008). Additionally, in Chinese culture, families are expected to cope with their relatives' illnesses, and so there might be a sense of shame when family members develop mental illness with carers becoming reluctant to ask for **professional support**. To compound this, it is well established that in any society a diagnosis of mental illness carries with it social stigma and discrimination (Chinese Mental Health Association 2011).

Therefore, in the past, it is possible that John might have failed to recognize the significance of his wife's psychological difficulties. He might also have been reluctant to ask for professional support or help from his children, and so mentioning this now may well signify that he is finding it difficult to cope, and that Daphne's psychological state is worsening.

It is also widely documented that most male carers tend to approach the caring role in a different way to female carers. Men tend to be more detached from the emotional aspects of caring and usually adopt a problem-centred approach to caring. While such a strategy can be useful in providing effective support, when a caring role is prolonged or practical approaches become unsustainable, anxiety and depression often result because the male carer feels he should cope and has failed to do so (Dahlberg et al. 2007).

4   **What support is available to carers and what are their rights?**

 The impact of caring has been comprehensively documented and the needs of carers extensively surveyed, yet many carers in similar situations to John still mention a lack of effective action and service provision to meet their needs (Jenkins 2004). In an attempt to rectify this situation, a number of strategies, policies and legislative measures have been published and implemented. These aim to ensure that care providers address carers' needs, and while these policies are not always specific to caring for people with mental health problems, it is clear that carers now have a number of rights, with care strategies in place to support them. These are summarized in Table 26.2.

Table 26.2 Carers' rights

Policies and legislative measures to support carers	Carers' rights
The Carer's (Recognition and services) Act (1995)	Gives individuals aged 16 years and over who provide 'substantial care on a regular basis' the right to request an assessment from social care agencies
The National Strategy Caring About Carers (1999)	Acknowledges the burden placed on carers and consists of three strategic elements: – the provision of information to carers, including a carers' charter – carer support; involving carers in planning and providing services – care, whereby the carers' own health needs are addressed

(Continued overleaf)

Table 26.2 Continued

Policies and legislative measures to support carers	Carers' rights
The Carers and Disabled Children's Act (2000)	Enables carers who provide (or intend to provide) a substantial amount of care on a regular basis to someone aged over 18 years to apply for a carers' assessment
The Carers (Equal opportunities) Act (2004)	Is intended to provide a firm foundation for better practice by local councils and the NHS. It builds on existing legislation and support for carers by placing a duty on local authorities to ensure that all carers know that they are entitled to an assessment of their needs; placing a duty on councils to consider a carer's outside interests (work, study or leisure) when carrying out an assessment; promoting better joint working between councils and the health service to ensure support for carers is delivered in a coherent manner
The Department of Health document: *Recognised, Valued and Supported: Next Steps for the Carers Strategy* (DoH 2010a)	Published in November 2010, this updates the 1999 national strategy by outlining the priorities for carers for the next four years. New funding will support four priority areas: – supporting those with caring responsibilities to identify themselves as carers at an early stage, recognizing the value of their contribution and involving them from the outset both in designing local care provision and in planning individual care packages – enabling those with caring responsibilities to fulfil their educational and employment potential – personalized support both for carers and those they support, enabling them to have a family and community life – supporting carers to remain mentally and physically well
The Department of Health document: *Carers and Personalisation: Improving Outcomes* (DoH 2010b)	Additional guidance published in November 2010 that included examples of how the principles of personalization have been adopted e.g. personal budgets. This document further highlights the importance of local partnerships and action plans
The Department of Health document: *No Health Without Mental Health: A Cross-Government Mental Health Outcomes Strategy for People of all Ages* (DoH 2011)	This mental health strategy integrated the revised carers' National Strategy priorities and requires professionals to develop a care plan for carers It acknowledges the importance of effectively supporting carers thereby enabling service users to remain at home It sets out six shared objectives to improve the mental health and well-being of UK citizens and to improve outcomes for people with mental health problems by providing high quality services

As a result of continuing assessment and discussion with John, the community mental health nurse identified a range of needs. These include the subjective and objective aspects of his caring role, and the cultural and gender features of his approach to the caring role.

5 **How might Mrs Chan's CPN use the Care Programme Approach (CPA) to meet John's needs and rights?**

A The CPA is the main assessment and care planning framework used in mental health practice and was introduced by the Department of Health in 1991 to ensure that people with a severe mental illness maintain contact with care services, receive an individualized assessment and an integrated, multi-disciplinary plan of care (Thompson and Strathdee 1997). The CPA was developed after a number of reports suggested that individuals with long-term mental health difficulties were not receiving the required help from mental health and social care providers (Reda 1994). To help overcome this, care plans have to be holistic, recovery-focused and structured to help the service user overcome social exclusion (DoH 2002).

Within the CPA all carers have the right to have their needs assessed and must receive their own written care plan, and have their needs reassessed annually (Rethink 2006). The principles of the 'carers' care plan' are the provision of information and advice, accessing respite services specifically for the carer, and making available additional services for the service user.

The needs of carers of people with mental health problems have been comprehensively researched and documented. Among the findings regarding the needs of carers is for someone to talk to, help with practical tasks, assistance with finances, support to enable them to take a break and effective care and treatment for the service user (Gregory et al. 2006). While Weinberg and Huxley (2000) also highlighted the value of **family support workers** as a counselling, listening, information and **advocacy** resource. Rethink (2006) reinforce the necessity of an assessment of carer needs, planned **respite care, direct payments**, local services and support groups, benefits awareness, time off and help during a crisis. Weinberg and Huxley (2000) further state that carers need a whole range of integrated services including emotional support, information and crisis advice. Also highlighted has been the requirement for practitioners to develop written care plans in partnership with carers and the need to support carers to develop self-help strategies (DoH 2002).

While the needs of carers have been clearly identified, often due to the time required of community practitioners to organize care packages for service users, carers' needs are often overlooked (DoH 2002). This is mainly because to develop a care plan for carers significantly increases the time spent on assessment and the subsequent implementation of care strategies. As a result, many carers such as John struggle to cope with the demands of their caring roles with only minimal support from the statutory agencies. The situation may well become worse in the near future with NHS Trusts and Local Authorities needing to make savings as a result of the Government's comprehensive spending review. In this respect carer organizations are expressing concern that support for carers will be reduced over the coming few years (Carers UK 2011).

6 **How might mental health promotion strategies be used to support John?**

A Mental health promotion is an integral part of carer support and is concerned with activities that improve the psychological well-being of all aspects of personal caring and include support to families and local communities (DoH 2001). To meet this requirement, two major strategies are advocated within this policy document:

- *Access to the community network and support for carers*: Close liaison by community practitioners with primary healthcare team members and multi-professional groups is needed to provide a package of care which effectively meets carer needs. Carers will continue to require a focus for access to the services available. The nursing role should therefore be proactive, forward thinking and planned, for example, organizing planned respite care, rather than waiting for a crisis to occur. There is also the scope for professionals to make a greater contribution to the support of carers, particularly by giving training in the skills which carers require.

* *Carer advocacy*: The growing awareness of carer burden requires that future planning of community-based care where a person with a mental health problem is supported by a carer needs to actively consider the needs of the carer. Mental health nurses can exert influence on behalf of carers by identifying these needs through care processes and the subsequent involvement of independent advocacy services but also by working with organizations which represent the interests of carers.

The mental health promotion strategies contained within this guidance (DoH 2001) are utilised in Table 26.3. These strategies could be used to meet John's needs in the ways described.

Table 26.3 Mental health promotion strategies

Mental health promotion strategy	Strategy description	Strategies to support John
Early intervention	Is concerned with targeting carers developing or experiencing their first problem	Carer's assessment of caring, physical, mental health, cultural and lifestyle needs
		A written care plan developed in partnership with John providing integrated, multi-agency care
		Psychological treatment and intervention to help alleviate his feelings of anxiety
		Refer Daphne for an early out-patients appointment to reassess her mental illness
		Involve John's family to help reduce his burden
Selected primary prevention	Refers to interventions designed to prevent a problem occurring	Information on the support services available to Daphne including carers' booklet, helplines and local support, e.g. Rethink
		Advice on financial matters, local carer support groups, internet-based information, Daphne's mental illness and support during a crisis
Secondary prevention	Is concerned with reducing the impact of problems through early interventions	Listening, counselling and emotional support
		Advise John on the practical aspects of caring to enable self-help strategies
		Provision of planned home respite
Tertiary prevention	Is concerned with reducing long-term problems	Act as an advocate and resource for John
		Investigate support provided by the Chinese mental health association

Effective support to carers can help to prevent in-patient admissions, and is consistent with recent developments in community-based mental health practice, such as **intensive home support** and relapse prevention (Healthcare Commission 2006). Carers have developed high levels of expertise from many years of experience, and so it is important to work in partnership with them to access their expertise and knowledge and enable empowerment and self-help (Rethink 2006). However, it is also important to acknowledge that due to the burden of caring, carers are at high risk of developing stress-related and mental health problems, and so it must be highlighted that any carers like John who experience such difficulties are themselves entitled to a CPA assessment (DoH 1996). With this in mind, the DoH (2002) guidance outlines innovative practice examples that go further than the strategies contained in the above planned support for John and are particularly aimed at emotional support. These include care plans that can provide 24-hour/7 days per week contact numbers, **family group conferencing,** psycho-social interventions, health education and carer training and targeted specialist care for ethnic groups (DoH 2002).

Mental health practice is subject to constant change, and so it is important to keep the needs of carers under constant review and for practitioners to ensure that carers' needs are assessed and care plans effectively implemented as required within the CPA and by current legislation. The forthcoming changes to the NHS will also require care professionals to embrace the principles of the Big Society and so become experts at utilizing the support to carers that is available in the independent and voluntary sectors and from primary care agencies.

REFERENCES

Barsky, A. J. (1992) Amplification, somatisation and the somatoform disorders, *Psychosomatics*, 33: 28–34.

Carers UK (2011) 4 out of 5 carers fear consequences of cuts to care services. Carers UK Web Page. Available at: http://www.carersuk.org/newsroom/item/2179-4-out-of-5-carers-fear-consequences-of-cuts-to-care-services (accessed 15 June 2011).

Cheng, A.T.A. (2001) Case definition and culture: are people all the same? *British Journal of Psychiatry*, 179: 1–3.

Chinese Mental Health Association (2011) Home web page: http://www.cmha.org.uk/(accessed 22 July 2011).

Dahlberg, L., Demack, S. and Bambra, C. (2007) Age and gender of informal carers: a population based study in the UK. *Health and Social Care in the Community*, 15(5): 439–45.

DoH (Department of Health) (1995) The Carer's (Recognition and Services) Act 1995. London: DoH.

DoH (Department of Health) (1996) *Reviewing the Care Programme Approach: A Consultation Document*. London: DoH.

DoH (Department of Health) (1999) *Caring about Carers*. London: DoH.

DoH (Department of Health) (2000) The Carers and Disabled Children's Act. London: DoH.

DoH (Department of Health) (2001) *Making It Happen: A Guide To Delivering Mental Health Promotion*. London: DoH.

DoH (Department of Health) (2002) *Developing Services for Carers and Families of People with Mental Illness*. London: DoH.

DoH (Department of Health) (2004) Carers (Equal Opportunities) Act 2004. London: DoH.

DoH (Department of Health) (2010a) *Recognised, Valued and Supported: Next Steps for the Carers Strategy*. London: DoH.

DoH (Department of Health) (2010b) *Carers and Personalisation*. London: DoH.

DoH (Department of Health) (2011) *No Health Without Mental Health: A Cross-Government Mental Health Outcomes Strategy for People of All Ages*. London: DoH.

Gregory, N., Collins-Atkins, C., Macpherson, R., Ford, S. and Palmer, A. (2006) Identifying the needs of carers in mental health services, *Nursing Times*, 102(17): 32–5.

Healthcare Commission (2006) *Improvement Review of Community Mental Health Services*. London: Healthcare Commission.

Jenkins, L. (2004) *The Ups and Downs of Bipolar Carers: An Investigation into the Coping Strategies and Needs of Bipolar Carers*. London: Mental Health Foundation.

Kung, W.W. and Lu, P. (2008) How symptom manifestations affect help seeking for mental health problems among Chinese Americans, *The Journal of Nervous and Mental Disease*, 196(1): 46–54.

Morris, K. (1991) Perceptions of burden in informal carers, *Journal of Mental Health Nursing*, 3(5): 245–52.

Reda, S. (1994) A study of psychiatric patients moved from hospital to community: baseline, six months and one year follow-up, *Journal of Mental Health*, 3(2): 249–55.

Rethink (2006) *Reach Out to Help Someone Cope with Severe Mental Illness*. London: Rethink.

Sin, J., Moone, N. and Wellman, N. (2005) Developing services for the carers of young adults with early-onset psychosis: listening to their experiences and needs, *Journal of Psychiatric & Mental Health Nursing*, 12(5): 589–97.

Thompson, K. and Strathdee, G. (1997) *The Care Programme Approach for Mental Health Teams*. London: Sainsbury Centre.

Weinberg, A. and Huxley, P. (2000) An evaluation of the impact of voluntary sector family support workers on the quality of life of carers of schizophrenia sufferers, *Journal of Mental Health* 9(5): 495–503.

WEB RESOURCES

Alzheimer's Society
http://www.alzheimers.org.uk/

Carer information
http://www.direct.gov.uk/en/CaringForSomeone/index.htm

Carers at the heart of 21st-century families and communities (Carers National Strategy)
http://www.dh.gov.uk/en/Publicationsandstatistics/Publications/PublicationsPolicy
AndGuidance/DH_085345

Carers UK web page
http://www.carersuk.org/

Chinese Mental Health Association
http://www.cmha.org.uk/

Department of Health carers page
http://www.dh.gov.uk/en/SocialCare/Carers/index.htm

The care programme approach
http://www.dh.gov.uk/en/Publicationsandstatistics/Publications/PublicationsPolicy
AndGuidance/DH_083647

Alcohol misuse in older adults
Nick Wrycraft

Ron is 78 years old. He spent much of his working life in the army and after leaving the service was employed as a security guard until his retirement. He greatly missed his work and had few other interests to occupy his time. Ron never married or had children but lived with his partner Alice whom he met after leaving the army. They had a quiet life although had a number of friends in the local area. Ron's main leisure activity was playing darts and pool at a local club for ex-servicemen where he used to meet and drink with friends.

Eighteen months ago, Alice died from a stroke. Since then Ron has became very low in mood, and stopped attending the club. Ron began drinking at home and not eating or caring for himself. A friend visited Ron and, concerned at the extent of his self-neglect, accompanied him to the GP who wrote to the community mental health team (CMHT) for older adults asking for an assessment of Ron's mental health due to his low mood and alcohol use.

The CMHT offered an assessment at their office with a community psychiatric nurse (CPN) and consultant psychiatrist. Ron attended with his friend and seemed very low in mood and looked dishevelled. He appeared to be disorientated and having problems remembering things although said this was due to his age. His breath smelt of alcohol, and Ron's friend explained that when he called for him this morning he was asleep on the couch, fully clothed.

When asked about his drinking, Ron said that he had always enjoyed the social contact. However, over the past year he stopped attending the club as his mood was low but also a number of younger people had joined and he found their behaviour rowdy and they insisted on playing loud music. Instead Ron began to drink at home in the daytime and eventually beginning in the mornings. He does not remember how much he drinks but accepts that once he starts he finds it hard to stop.

Ron said that Alice used to insist on doing all of the housework and cleaning and even dealt with their finances. Since her death, he has struggled to maintain the home and is worried about money. He believes that he owes money to the utility companies and has stopped opening his mail. Ron said that he associated drinking with enjoyable times and uses it as a way of 'forgetting about my worries'.

1   **Is alcohol misuse common among older adults?**

A   Of all of the alcohol-related hospital admissions to hospital in the NHS in 2009, over half were for people over 60 years of age, with causes ranging from falls to liver damage due to alcohol, while the proportion of older people in the UK experiencing health issues related to alcohol has increased (Alcohol Issues 2010; NCCMH 2011; RCP 2010).

Together with the expectation of people living longer the effects of alcohol on the physical and mental health of older adults and the burden on the health services is likely to continue to rise. The government has issued guidance on harmful drinking for younger adults although these focus on the harm of excessive intake and public order issues (DoH 2007; NCCMH 2011; NICE 2010). Instead it has been suggested that guidance for alcohol misuse among older adults is much needed, as problems seem to occur among this age group for different reasons than younger people. Among these are:

- Social exclusion, as there is a limited provision of social opportunities for older people within society leading to inactivity and boredom.
- The effects of significant life changes which people in this age group often experience, such as ill health and bereavement.
- Economic problems due to people often living on fixed and limited incomes and drinking to forget problems.
- Reduced physical **tolerance** to the effects of alcohol as we grow older, meaning that older people are more susceptible to the effects of alcohol.

(Ward et al. 2008)

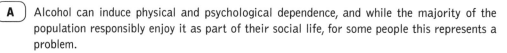

2   **What are the physical and psychological health-related risks for older adults regarding alcohol misuse?**

A   Alcohol can induce physical and psychological dependence, and while the majority of the population responsibly enjoy it as part of their social life, for some people this represents a problem.

Physically:

- As we grow older, often hearing and vision are less acute, while alcohol has the potential to impair coordination and the ability to judge distances, and may predispose older adults who drink to falls or accidents (Alcohol Issues 2010).
- As we age, our bodies slow down and our organs process food and liquid more slowly and less efficiently. Significantly our level of tolerance to alcohol also becomes less, meaning that the person may experience a greater physical and psychological response to smaller amounts of alcohol. Recent guidance suggests that revised safe drinking limits for older people might be helpful (NCCMH 2011).
- Alcohol is also a toxin which the body works hard to expel, and processing it is a complex physiological function:
  - initially alcohol is absorbed in the gut;
  - then processed in the liver and kidneys;
  - before being expelled through urine, breath or perspiration.

Therefore there is great potential for alcohol to contribute to health problems in a range of areas of the person's physical functioning.

Alcohol is known to cause or worsen the effects of other pre-existent health problems. For example:

- diabetes;
- high blood pressure (hypertension);
- heart disease.

Psychologically: After being consumed, alcohol is rapidly absorbed into the bloodstream, permeates the blood–brain barrier and influences our psychological functioning. Alcohol can make people more sociable, but can also affect judgement and cause people to be more uninhibited, and in some cases prone to uncharacteristic aggression, risky behaviour or carrying out impulsive acts. Although people often drink when they are low in mood, alcohol is a depressant, and likely to compound these feelings. There is also evidence that alcohol can cause cognitive impairment, for example Wernicke–Korsakoff syndrome and other dementia-type illnesses.

3 **What reasons might account for Ron's alcohol misuse?**

A The experiences which people can undergo in later life can create circumstances which predispose them to experiencing problems with alcohol (Ward et al. 2008):

- Ron has stopped going to the club which he used to frequent. In contrast with other cultures where older people are often venerated, our society tends to focus on younger people which often leads to older people experiencing social exclusion. Frequently older people feel vulnerable in social settings, and even reluctant to go out at night which can limit social opportunities, and lead to isolation, a lower quality of life and impact on mood and mental well-being (Ward et al. 2008).
- Ron missed his work and did not have other interests. Retirement can often lead to a sense of loss of identity, and the absence of a role and purpose, and in Ron's case he does not have a family or a range of interests and social relationships which might fill this void. It is possible that Ron drinks because he feels bored and under-occupied.
- Ron, like many older people, has experienced bereavement and lacks the close and supportive links which might be provided by a family network.
- Furthermore, within the relationship Alice performed many of the domestic tasks and paid all of the bills. Ron now has to perform tasks in which he does not feel confident and lacks support, which perhaps leads him to drink in order to mask his worries.

The Institute of Alcohol Studies (IAS) (2010) identifies several categories of alcohol misuse among older people:

- **Early onset** – where the person has experienced a drinking problem in earlier life which has continued.
- **Late onset** – as a reaction to a life event.
- **Binge drinkers** – who intermittently intake high levels of alcohol.

4 **Which of the above apply to Ron?**

A Early onset; it is possible that he has been an ongoing high user of alcohol, which means that he is within the early onset category. However, he feels that his problem has only begun recently in response to his bereavement and life circumstances and might also have developed a late onset problem.

ASSESSMENT

There are a number of different assessment tools for alcohol use. However, among the factors which might identify whether the person has a problem with alcohol are:

- drinking on most or all days of the week;
- consuming a large amount of alcohol in one sitting;
- not being able to stop drinking;
- needing to drink in the morning;
- feeling guilty after drinking;
- unable to remember events due to drinking;
- having an accident as a result of drinking;
- another person either family or friend has been concerned about the person's drinking;
- drinking alone or hiding alcohol;

(Babor et al. 2001)

Ron falls into a **high risk drinking** category as:

- he drinks every day;
- he drinks in the morning;
- he is unable to stop drinking once he has started;
- he is unable to remember events due to drinking;
- he has a friend who has become concerned;
- he drinks alone.

5 **What interventions might help Ron?**

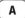

- A full physical health check was carried out. Ron was fortunate as his physical health was found to be generally good except for a deficiency in **vitamin B** which is very common among people who are high alcohol users. Ron was prescribed vitamin B **(thiamine)**.
- The psychiatrist suggested to Ron that he might wish to take anti-depressant medication to improve his mood. While it is generally recommended not to drink when taking prescribed medication, some anti-depressants can be taken when the person drinks alcohol (NHS Choices 2010). Ron was sceptical and concerned that these might make him drowsy and lethargic. However, the psychiatrist suggested that Ron's progress could be monitored, and if he experienced side effects, the medication could be reviewed.
  Ron agreed for a community psychiatric nurse (CPN) to visit him at home each week to provide psychological support and to work with him to achieve his goals.

Ron's health would benefit from stopping his excessive use of alcohol. However, this depends upon the level of motivation which he has to stop drinking. While Ron was willing to accept help, he felt that he could not promise to stop drinking.

Although Ron's alcohol misuse might be regarded as the most important issue, it is important that Ron and the CPN have an equal relationship based on trust, confidence and mutual collaboration. Often social stereotyping leads to people who misuse alcohol being labelled which can create an expectation within the person that they will be judged negatively and further damage self-esteem and confidence. Therefore, the CPN needs to adopt an approach which does not reflect any preconceptions yet which is still genuine.

At their first meeting the CPN suggested that Ron might like to keep a **drinking diary** (Table 27.1) which could be discussed each week. They then asked Ron what issues he wished to work on first. The CPN's approach empowered Ron in three respects:

1 The drinking diary enables Ron to appraise and reflect upon the evidence of his behaviour choices.
2 Ron is identifying the priorities on which to work which places him in control of his own therapeutic work.
3 Meaningful change to patterns of behaviour such as Ron's drinking requires significant commitment. Therefore it is preferable for Ron to choose whether this is a priority issue for him.

The issues on which Ron wished to work were:

* finances;
* increasing his level of activity.

Table 27.1 A drinking diary

Day	Amount and type of alcohol	Time started and time ended	Who was I with?	Where was I?	Number of units	Cost £	Thoughts/ feelings
Monday		Started: Ended:					
Tuesday		Started: Ended:					
Wednesday		Started: Ended:					
Thursday		Started: Ended:					
Friday		Started Ended:					
Saturday		Started: Ended:					
Sunday		Started: Ended:					

Source: Adapted from Kipping (2005).

Finances: The CPN discussed Ron's finances with him and arranged for a meeting with a voluntary financial advisor. The advisor helped him understand his financial circumstances better and make a plan for the payment of his bills on an ongoing basis. To Ron's surprise, his financial situation was much better than he anticipated, which removed much of his worry. However, he still tended to be reluctant to deal with his finances and to be frugal with his money.

Increased level of activity: Ron said that he wanted to be more active and to have more routine and structure to his day. The CPN suggested that Ron might find activity scheduling useful, and explained how this technique functions. Activity scheduling helps the person to manage their motivation, and set goals and achieve tasks (see Table 8.1 on p. 68). The person initially considers activities in several different categories, which include:

- pleasurable activities;
- activities which give a sense of achievement;
- activities which keep the person physically active;
- social activities;
- routine activities.

In Ron's case, watching sport was an activity which gave him pleasure and in discussion with the CPN he decided to purchase a subscription to a television sports channel. In contrast, Ron identified cooking as a routine activity which he did not enjoy and of which he had little experience. Therefore, Ron managed his motivation so that the necessary activity of preparing his tea was then followed with the pleasure of being able to watch sport afterwards. As this technique is for use with people working on their motivation in the initial stages of activity scheduling, it is best for the person to work with the healthcare practitioner in order to gain support.

Ron next identified that the task of going out and being among other people would give him a sense of achievement. This also fulfilled the criteria of physical and social activity yet also represented a challenge as he had lost confidence and experienced significant anxiety about going out. Ron set himself a target of going out twice a week to walk to his friends' house to meet up with them. Also he decided to go to the local supermarket once a week to do his shopping and initiate conversation with the person on the checkout.

After several weeks Ron had some success meeting his goals. However, he felt he lacked skills in cooking and knowledge of what to eat for a healthy diet and felt that he needed more activities to fill his time. Building on Ron's gaining confidence in going out, with his agreement, the CPN arranged for Ron to attend a local day hospital two days a week, where he attended cooking groups and gained knowledge of nutrition and received a lunchtime meal. At the day hospital Ron's memory was assessed, and while he appeared to be forgetful, his memory was not significantly impaired. It was agreed that the day hospital staff and the CPN would monitor Ron's memory and it would be assessed on a six-monthly basis or more frequently if it was felt to be deteriorating.

During each visit the CPN asked Ron about his drinking yet always in a casual manner, and although he continued to drink significant amounts, the CPN did not pass judgement on Ron's reply to avoid impacting on his self-esteem and potentially undermining the therapeutic relationship. The CPN also discussed the drinking diaries on each visit with Ron. Initially these were filled out incompletely; however, the detail increased following Ron's success with the activity scheduling, and as Ron became more acquainted with completing the forms. Ron and the CPN noticed that when he attended the day hospital or had activities to occupy his day, he drank less. This understanding reinforced Ron's perception that he drank more when he had less to do out of boredom. Furthermore, Ron was surprised at the amount of money he spent on alcohol and decided to reduce this figure and to only drink after a certain time in the evening. In order to further fill his days Ron began attending groups at his local community centre and library, and to go out for at least a few hours each day and through starting to drink later has reduced his alcohol intake.

Due to the physically and psychologically dependence-inducing effects of alcohol making relapse a high possibility, many therapeutic approaches suggest the need for abstinence (NCCMH 2011). Due to Ron reducing rather than abstaining, there is a possibility of his alcohol use increasing suddenly, and at times he has experienced relapse. In reviewing the drinking diaries, it was noticed that often these instances occur where he experiences a misfortune or his mood lowers and the increased consumption continues for several days before returning to the previous level. Together with the CPN Ron devised a relapse prevention plan to consider how he manages setbacks and reversals, and which will help him to minimize the harmful effects when his alcohol intake does increase.

CONCLUSION

Changing established behaviours can be challenging and it is often advisable to build confidence and to improve other areas of life first before focusing on what might be perceived as the most significant problem. Making sustainable change needs to be achieved in gradual and incremental steps. However, this is difficult for people such as Ron who lack the support of a family and supportive social network which might help his motivation, and he has also experienced social exclusion similar to that of many older people. While Ron has demonstrated considerable coping resources in making progress, his CPN needs to carefully support him in maintaining the structure he has established in his life and which has helped him to reduce his drinking. It is necessary for Ron to continue to engage in other rewarding alternative activities in order to maintain his progress.

REFERENCES

Alcohol Issues (2010) Alcohol and the older person. Available at: http://www.alcoholissues.co.uk/alcohol-older-person.html (accessed 10 December 2010).

Babor, T.F., Higgins-Biddle, J.C, Saunders, J.B. and Monteiro, M.G. (2001) *Audit: The Alcohol Use Disorders Identification Test: Guidelines for Use in Primary Care*, 2nd edn. Geneva: World Health Organization.

BBC (n.d.) *Headroom* Well Being Guide, Activity scheduling: The fabulous four. Available at: http://downloads.bbc.co.uk/headroom/cbt/activity_scheduling.pdf (accessed 25 October 2011).

DoH (Department of Health) (2007) *Safe, Sensible, Social: The Next Steps in the National Alcohol Strategy*. London: DoH.

Institute of Alcohol Studies (2010) *Alcohol and the Elderly: IAS Factsheet*. Available at: http://www.ias.org.uk (accessed 10 December 2010).

Kipping, C. (2005) The person who misuses drugs or alcohol, in N. Norman and I. Ryne (eds) *The Art and Science of Mental Health Nursing: A Textbook of Principles and Practice.* Maidenhead: McGraw-Hill, pp. 481–518.

Lister, S. (2009) Growing problems of alcohol abuse among elderly uncovered, *The Times & The Sunday Times.* Available at: http://business.timesonline.co.uk/tol/business/industry_sectors/health/article6701795.ece (accessed 28 December 2010).

Mental Health Foundation (2006) *Cheers? Understanding the Relationship Between Alcohol and Mental Health.* London: The Mental Health Foundation.

NCCMH (National Collaborating Centre for Mental Health) (2011) *Alcohol-Use Disorders: The NICE Guidelines on Diagnosis, Assessment and Management of Harmful Drinking and Alcohol Dependence.* National Clinical Practice Guideline 115. London: The British Psychological Society and The Royal College of Psychiatrists.

NHS Choices (2010) Can I drink alcohol if I'm taking antidepressants? Available at: http://www.nhs.uk/chq/Pages/863.aspx?CategoryID=73&SubCategoryID=103(accessed 24 October 2011).

NICE (National Institute for Health and Clinical Excellence) (2008) *Occupational Therapy Interventions and Physical Activity to Promote the Mental Wellbeing of Older People in Primary and Residential Care.* London: NICE.

NICE (National Institute for Health and Clinical Excellence) (2010) *Alcohol Use Disorders: Preventing the Development of Hazardous and Harmful Drinking.* London: NICE.

RCP (Royal College of Psychiatrists) (2010) *Alcohol and Older People.* Available at: http://www.rcpsych.ac.uk/mentalhealthinfoforall/problems/alcoholanddrugs/alcoholandolderpeople.aspx (accessed 28 January 2010).

Ward, L., Barnes, M. and Gahagen, B. (2008) *Cheers?!A Project about Older People and Alcohol.* Brighton: University of Brighton.

Glossary

Abandonment: Abandonment is concerned with the feelings and experiences we encounter when we lose somebody or their affection, approval, protection, or friendship. It is about the loss of love itself, that crucial loss of connectedness to another person, or object of our affection. Abandonment can also be about the events that cause that crucial loss of connectedness. These experiences can be real, feared or imagined.

Active listening: Demonstrating to the person speaking that we are listening through gesture, speaking and facial expression.

Activity scheduling: Recording activity which the person carries out. Often this is helpful where the person lacks motivation by identifying tasks which the person has prioritized and then providing a record to evidence achievement which offers structure and helps with the setting of goals.

Acute stress disorder: The development of features of generic anxiety together with dissociation and other symptoms generally within a brief interval of exposure to an extreme source of stress.

Admiral nurses: Specialist mental health nurses who use a range of interventions to support people with dementia and their families in the community.

Advocacy: An integral part of a healthcare professional's code of conduct which requires professionals to work within the best interests of the service user and ensure that their views are heard and respected.

Affect: Subjectively experienced emotions which can be observed.

Affective disorder: Problems with emotions which affect the person's everyday functioning.

Agenda: Forms the agreement on which parties meet and consists of all of the issues which will be discussed. Keeping to the agenda prevents the discussion drifting and failing to address the shared issues of concern.

Akathisia: Feeling of inner restlessness and need to move and inability to remain still.

Alcohol dependence: The World Health Organization (WHO 2001) defines alcohol dependence as behavioural, physiological and psychological features after repeated use of alcohol. Behaviourally and psychologically, these include:
- a significant desire to consume alcohol;
- the inability to control drinking;
- preoccupation with alcohol over other activities and obligations;
- persistence with drinking in spite of harmful consequences.

Physical features are:
- developing tolerance to larger amounts of alcohol;
- experiencing symptoms of withdrawal when not drinking.

All or nothing thinking: A thinking style based on the premise that if the person does not succeed completely, then they have failed and there is nothing between these criteria.

Alogia (poverty of speech): The individual finds it difficult to sustain fluent conversation, and to give additional or unprompted information; conversation can be monosyllabic or repetitive.

Amenorrhea: The loss of the menstrual cycle.

Amyloid plaques: Characteristic of Alzheimer's disease, they accumulate between nerve cells. These would usually be broken down and eliminated but in Alzheimer's disease fragments accumulate to form hard, insoluble plaques.

Anhedonia (blunt affect): This is when the individual experiences a reduction in pleasure, emotion and enjoyment in everyday life.

Anti-cholinesterase: A brain chemical that prevents the cholinesterase enzyme from breaking down acetylcholine. The three acetylcholinesterase inhibitor drugs are:

- Aricept (donepezil hydrochloride)
- Exelon (rivastigmine)
- Reminyl (galantamine).

Anti-depressant medication: Commonly prescribed medications for depression include monoamine oxidase inhibitors (MAOIs), selective serotonin reuptake inhibitors (SSRIs) and tricyclics.

Antipsychotic medications: A group of medications that work on specific receptors of the brain; they are also known as neuroleptics and are sometimes referred to as major tranquillizers, although this is a misleading term. They are available in an oral and depot (long-lasting) injection preparation and are used to treat a wide variety of mental illnesses. They are often referred to as typical anti-psychotics and atypical anti-psychotics. The typical anti-psychotics are an older group for example, haloperidol and chlorpromazine, and the atypical antipsychotics are the newer anti-psychotics and include olanzapine, quetiapine and aripiprazole. Each drug has its own specific benefit and can cause a range of the unwanted side effects ranging from sedation to weight gain.

Arrhythmia: Irregular heartbeat.

Assertive outreach: Providing ongoing support for people with long-term severe and enduring mental health problems.

Assessment: A process of gathering information to explore the person's experience and to find out about what is their reality. Specific assessment tools might also be used as appropriate to ascertain further information and measure the person's problems as appropriate and consistent with their level of engagement and collaboration.

Assistive technology: A system that enables an individual to perform an activity they would not otherwise be able to undertake. This includes equipment to help with speaking, hearing, eyesight, moving, memory and cognition. Tools include calendar clocks, touch lamps and satellite navigation systems to help find a lost person.

Attachment: An infant activates the attachment process by seeking proximity to the primary caregivers to feel more secure in their presence. Attachment refers to the emotional bonds in early infancy. Importance is placed on the quality of early parent–child relationships on child mental health as this relationship provides the building blocks not just for their relationship but the child's overall emotional development. The attachment system is relevant across the age range, including adulthood.

Avoidance: A defence mechanism whereby the person carries out other activities to avoid distressing memories.

Avoiding: Not confronting a problem.

Behaviour: Actions or responses to stimuli.

Behavioural experiment: Carrying out an activity to overcome a fear. Often this involves assessing the level of fear or discomfort before and after the activity.

Behavioural rehearsal: Role play replicating situations or relationships where the person finds explaining their feelings difficult.

Benzodiazepines: Part of the hypnotic and anxiolytic group of drugs. Their purpose is to help alleviate anxiety, insomnia and to aid muscle relaxation.

Binge drinking: Intermittent consumption of a large amount of alcohol.

Binging: Process by which an individual will consume a very high number of calories in a single sitting, often using high fat content foods and carried out alone and in secret.

Bipolar disorder: Formerly known as manic depression and characterized by the occurrence of at least one episode of what is called mania or hypomania. Bipolar disorder involves cycles of high and low extremes of mood which vary from the person's norm. These feelings vary between, at one extreme, low mood and features which are consistent with clinical depression, while, at the other, experiencing overt elation and happiness, although the person may also be angry or irritable. There are two levels of severity of bipolar disorder which are defined below.

Bipolar I disorder: Defined by manic or mixed episodes lasting at least seven days, or by manic symptoms so severe the person needs immediate hospital care. The person usually also has depressive episodes, typically lasting at least two weeks. Mania is unique to bipolar I disorder, and the symptoms of mania or depression are a major change from the person's normal behaviour.

Bipolar II disorder: Defined by a pattern of depressive episodes shifting back and forth with hypomanic episodes, but the occurrence of no manic or mixed episodes. Hypomania is characteristic of bipolar II. The difference between the two types of bipolar disorder depends on the severity of the elevation of mood, with mania being unique to bipolar I disorder and hypomania characteristic of bipolar II disorder.

Body dysmorphic disorder (BDD): DSM-IV-TR defines body dysmorphic disorder as follows:

A Preoccupation with an imagined defect in appearance. If a slight physical anomaly is present, the person's concern is markedly excessive.

B The preoccupation causes clinically significant distress or impairment in social, occupational, or other important areas of functioning.

C The preoccupation is not better accounted for by another mental disorder (e.g. dissatisfaction with body shape and size in anorexia nervosa).

Body Mass Index (BMI): An indication of ideal weight based on age and height.

Borderline personality disorder: Characterized by people having problems forming and maintaining appropriate and effective relationships with others, and unstable or impaired self-image beginning in childhood or adolescence. It is evident in a number of different contexts in the person's life, including close personal relationships, social network, education, occupation and employment, housing and finances. Characteristic of people with borderline personality disorder is the experience of repeated crises in various areas of their lives. Often these difficulties are also experienced regarding personal image and identity, and sense of values, principles and beliefs.

Boundaries: Establishing mutual expectations and goals. Within a therapeutic relationship, the focus is on promoting the mental well-being of the person with the nurse advocating on their behalf and supporting the person's empowerment and optimal capacity for self-determination.

Bullying: A form of aggressive behaviour intended to injure, insult, humiliate or undermine a person's dignity, confidence and self-esteem, which is often persistent and focused. Often bullying involves an imbalance of power with the aggressor in an empowered role either being senior in rank, physically more powerful or influential socially and is frequently focused on ethnicity, gender, religion, sexuality or ability. Bullying can be physical, psychological or emotional abuse and often takes the form of coercion or intimidation.

CAMHS: Child and Adolescent Mental Health Services.

CAMHS Tiered approach: 'The tiered model is now generally accepted as the way to describe and understand C A M H S.' (Richardson and Wyatt 2010: 10).

Tier 1 = G Ps, school nurses, health visitors.

Tiers 2 and 3 = A more specialized service offered by individual professionals (Tier 2) or via multi-disciplinary teams of nurses, psychologists, psychotherapists, psychiatrists and occupational therapists (Tier 3). Tiers 2 and 3 should operate in close collaboration, ideally from the same geographic base.

Tier 4 = Specialist services such as in-patient psychiatric care.

Care coordinator: A mental health professional who is appointed for a service user under the Care Programme Approach; this is a process for care delivery and review that has been part of mental health services since 1991. It has been reviewed and refocused, and it ensures the identification of a key worker/care coordinator for appropriate service users, and that they are responsible for a number of things, including overseeing the process, liaising, risk assessment and planning, and a point of contact.

Care Programme Approach (CPA): The C PA is the National Framework which provides a unified system of assessment, documentation of care and coordination by one named healthcare professional in each person's care. It was introduced as a result of the Community Care Act (1990)

Carer: A generic term that can be used to describe either formal carers, or people who are employed to care, or informal carers which refers to families, friends and neighbours. It is important that professionals avoid generalized assumptions about who are carers, and clarify with service users and significant others, their roles and relationships. Professionals also need to recognize that caring relationships may change over time.

Carers assessment: Carers have the right to an assessment of their needs. The outcome of this should be a collaborative and focused plan detailing named contacts, actions, a crisis plan which also includes consideration of when this occurs outside of working hours, and timescales for the delivery of services. It should also, where possible, link with the Care Programme Approach (C PA) of the person supported.

Carers support: Support offered to carers. The type and level of which will depend on the individualized need identified in assessment.

Catastrophic thoughts: Often known as 'all or nothing' thinking, whereby the person thinks of the worst possible outcome for an event.

Central nervous system (CNS): Located in the brain and spinal cord and containing billions of cells, or neurons which use chemical messengers called neurotransmitters to increase or reduce activity in other neurons.

Child and Adolescent Mental Health Services (CAMHS): A service for children with mental health problems.

Citalopram: A selective serotonin reuptake inhibitor (SSRI) anti-depressant medication.

Class A drug: The most powerful and regulated classification of controlled drugs. These include: opiates (heroin), cocaine, crack cocaine, ecstasy, LSD, psilocybin (magic mushrooms).

Class B drug: The second most powerful and regulated classification of controlled drugs including: amphetamine (Class A if prepared for injecting), cannabis, mephedrone.

Class C drug: The third and lowest band of regulated and controlled drugs, including: benzo-diazepines (unless prescribed), ketamine, anabolic steroids, GHB.

Closed questions: Questions with a fixed range of response, for example, those with only a 'yes' or 'no' answer.

Code of professional conduct: A set of guiding principles and expectations that are considered binding when a person agrees to become a member of a particular professional group.

Cognitions: How we know information, which is arrived at through processes including awareness, intuition, judgement and perception.

Cognitive behavioural therapy (CBT): A structured and time-limited psychological therapy which aims to help the person develop practical ways of working with their problem. CBT considers how the person feels in response to events and to consider their thoughts (cognitions) and feelings and the effects these have on their behaviour. CBT combines cognitive and behavioural approaches in helping the person develop practical strategies for dealing with problems.

Cognitive difficulties: Can occur in schizophrenia and the individual may find it hard to concentrate, to make decisions or plan and sustain activities and may experience impaired memory.

Cognitive stimulation therapy: A programme of group activities for people with dementia based on the principles of reality orientation.

Comforting data log: Monitoring thoughts for thoughts which are positive and provide comfort.

Communication: Speech, signs or actions which are used to transmit information to another party.

Community Mental Health Team (CMHT): Community-based multi-disciplinary teams working within specialist mental health services who work with people with a range of different mental health problems.

Community psychiatric nurse (CPN): A nurse who works with people in the community. Their functions are wide and varied but include:
- providing support in all aspects of the person's functioning;
- ongoing therapeutic input;
- supporting carers and significant others;
- medication monitoring;
- administering medication.

Co-morbidity: The coexistence of two or more disorders or diseases.

Compensatory behaviours: The individual will attempt to counteract their binge in a number of ways. These can include vomiting, using laxatives and diuretics or excessive exercising.

Complex phobias: A phobia concerning a particular circumstance or situation; examples include agoraphobia.

Compulsions: Repetitive behaviours or mental acts which the person feels compelled to perform in connection with their obsessive thoughts in order to reduce distress, or to prevent a feared outcome. Compulsive acts are not experienced as pleasurable, with many people feeling shame or guilt and a sense of a loss of self-determination in performing these actions.

Computerized CBT (CCBT): A computer programme which carries out CBT interventions with the person.

Conduct disorder: Conduct disorder is recognized in DSM-IV-TR (APA 2000). It is defined, in summary, as:

A repetitive and persistent pattern of behaviour in which the basic rights of others or major age-appropriate societal norms or rules are violated, as manifested by the presence of three (or more) of the following criteria in the past 12 months, with at least one criterion present in the past 6 months:

Aggression to people and animals; destruction of property; deceitfulness or theft; serious violations of rules.

The disturbance in behaviour causes clinically significant impairment in social, academic, or occupational functioning.

If the individual is aged 18 years or older, criteria are not met for Antisocial Personality Disorder.

Confabulation: The production of false memories which are either memories for events that never happened or memories of real events that occurred at a different time.

Coping mechanism: An adaptation to stress based on conscious or unconscious choice and which enhances control over behaviour or provides psychological comfort.

Core beliefs: Fundamental beliefs about the nature of the world which are often active in maintaining problems.

Counselling: Two people form a therapeutic relationship by formally meeting at an arranged time and place. The client uses the meeting space to discuss issues of concern and to make sense of their feelings. The trained counsellor listens, acknowledges the concerns, and offers support to enable the client to make changes.

Couple counselling: This is for two persons who have formed an intimate relationship. The couple work is carried out with a trained therapist exploring communication issues, commitments, roles, and responsibilities. Respect, honesty and mutual support are important.

Covert compulsions: Non-visible compulsions often in the form of mental acts.

Criminal Justice and Court diversion: Liaising with the Courts to provide mental health assessments and reports for people in the Criminal Justice system.

Crisis: Crisis is a perception or experiencing of an event or situation as an intolerable difficulty that exceeds the person's current resources and coping mechanisms. In times of crisis people tend to be dependent, more open to suggestion and advice than they usually are. Crisis intervention aims to capitalize on this psychological state to achieve the maximum impact on the individual and his family with the maximum of medical intervention.

Crisis Resolution and Home Treatment (CRHT): The CRHT is an example of a range of community-based mental health services which were introduced as a result of the *National Service Framework for Mental Health* (DoH 1999) and aims to work with people undergoing crisis in their own homes. The rationale for this initiative was to reconfigure services to allow people with mental health problems to reside in the community, to reduce the trauma of in-patient admission and to promote rehabilitation by removing the need for service users to reorientate to their homes when they are discharged from in-patient units.

Day hospital: A clinical area staffed by nurses, people from other healthcare disciplines and unqualified staff. People attend for programmes of planned therapeutic programmes which form part of an agreed plan of care. Often these involve themed groups or activities. Day hospitals provide care which has a specific therapeutic focus with attendance for a limited time and is regularly reviewed.

Delusions: Specific thought disorders that were once described as fixed false belief. They are now thought to be based in a distorted or exaggerated reality, that is false within the cultural context of the individual and open to challenging, testing and modifying.

Dementia cafés: Provide an informal meeting point for carers and individuals with dementia to meet others and to obtain information and support from mental health workers.

Dental erosion: The process by which an individual loses the enamel on their teeth due to the repeated introduction of stomach acid into the mouth through self-induced vomiting.

Depressants: Act on the CNS to decrease brain activity and can make the user feel drowsy and calm. They also help to reduce pain.

Depression: An affective disorder characterized by the loss of enjoyment of life, and evident in the form of pervasive low mood, and a number of other features which are a significant alteration from the person's normal functioning. These features include behavioural, cognitive, emotional and physical factors (APA 2000; NCCMH 2011). See also Appendix in Case study 2.

Detoxification: The process of stopping using a substance.

Developmental disorder: Any problem that occurs during a child's development that hinders the child's physical or psychological development. Developmental disorders include autistic spectrum disorder, attention deficit and hyperactivity disorder, Tourette's syndrome and problems in toileting such as encopresis (problems with bowel control) and enuresis (problems with bladder control).

Developmental history: A detailed history of the physical and emotional development of an individual, including their mother's health during pregnancy. Other significant factors to consider as part of a developmental history are details of the individual's birth (particularly any birth trauma), attachment to the primary caregiver, feeding and sleeping patterns, and milestones such as sitting, crawling, talking and walking.

Dialectic behavioural therapy (DBT): DBT is a treatment designed for people with borderline personality disorder, particularly those with suicidal behaviour. DBT aims to help people with BPD to validate their emotions and behaviours, examine those behaviours and emotions that have a negative impact on their lives, and make a conscious effort to bring about positive changes.

Diazepam: A benzodiazepine usually given for the short-term alleviation of anxiety due to the potential for the person to develop a physical and or psychological dependence, even based on brief use.

Direct payments: Funds that are made available to carers or service users by local authorities to enable them to purchase services from a range of health or social care agencies. This enables personal choice and individualized care.

Disordered thoughts: Statements which are based on delusions or hallucinations.

Dissociative symptoms: Feelings that your body does not quite belong to you or is disconnected from you or feelings that you are disconnected from the world around you or 'spaced out'.

Dopamine: A chemical found in the brain that acts as a neurotransmitter, that is, it acts to transmit messages between nerve cells (neurons) in the brain. Dopamine is important in the regulation of emotion and physical movement. Shortage of dopamine is associated with Parkinson's disease.

Drinking diary: A structured record of the person's alcohol intake. The information which is collected might vary but commonly identifies the amount consumed and type, how long the drinking carried on for, when, where and who the person was with, and the cost.

DSM-IV: *The Diagnostic and Statistical Manual of Mental Disorders,* published by the American Psychiatric Association. It is revised regularly. DSM-IV is used by many health professionals to help them to arrive at a diagnosis.

Dysphoria: An emotional state marked by anxiety, depression and dissatisfaction.

Early Intervention in Psychosis (EiP): To facilitate rapid access to services for younger adults experiencing acute mental health problems.

Early onset drinking: Where a person has a pre-existent alcohol problem which endures into later life.

Electroconvulsive therapy (ECT): A treatment whereby an electrical current is passed through the brain with the intention of inducing a seizure. ECT is only used where other treatment options have not been successful and the person's quality of life and functioning are severely affected. Most often, ECT is used for people with acute depression. There is no evidence base to support the use of this intervention although some people report beneficial improvements in mood; however, some people also report ongoing memory impairment afterwards.

Emetophobia: A persistent, extreme and disproportionate concern about vomiting, either of self or other people. It may be linked to worries over losing control or of others finding the person repulsive. The person becomes preoccupied with vomiting to the extent it dominates their life and prevents them carrying out everyday activities of living. As a result, the person carries out safety behaviours to avoid situations which may place them in a situation which may make them likely to be in the presence of people who might vomit.

Emotion: The element of consciousness which involves feeling and is present without conscious effort.

Engagement: Demonstrating empathy and understanding and allowing self-efficacy through mutual respect and support.

Erikson's life stage theory: Suggests that in order to develop and progress through life there are eight challenges which need to be successfully negotiated in order to progress to the next. See Case study 21.

Evaluation: The final stage of a cycle commonly referred to by the acronym APIE. This stands for Assessment, Planning, Implementation and Evaluation. Evaluation identifies whether intended goals have been met through care interventions. The cycle is continuously repeated and fundamental to the approach used by healthcare professionals in applying an evidence-based and person-centred approach.

Exposure: Confronting the feared situation or phenomena.

Exposure and Response Prevention (ERP): The treatment recommended for use with people experiencing OCD by the NICE guidance (2005). This is a behaviourally based intervention and involves the person facing their feared situation without employing their safety behaviours.

Expressed emotion: Present within three attitudes displayed by family members of a person with a mental health problem. These are: hostile, critical and over-involved.

Family-based work: The context of the family is vital to understanding the young person's world and problems. The parents are partners in the care of young people. In family meetings, all family members' perspectives are listened to, patterns of relating and behavioural patterns unfold, insight into the difficulties emerge and then change can occur. This approach is used in conjunction with other interventions.

Family group conferencing: A therapeutic technique to improve communication and problem solving within families by bringing the family unit together. This approach is based on the assumption that difficulties can only be resolved by involving all key family members.

Family sculpting: A creative exercise using artistic media such as paint or clay. The family is invited to construct a representation of family relationships, then to experiment by making changes, for example, by moving clay figures or drawings to produce a new image. The aim is 'to represent family relationships and positions as the sculptor sees it at present. To explore possible changes by moving the figures around' (Asen and Scholz 2010: 65).

Family support workers: Non-professionally trained care staff who provide time-limited but intensive support to families who are finding it difficult to cope. Such workers have usually undertaken national vocational qualifications in care and so are able to implement a range of supportive measures.

Fine motor skills: Involve the development of groups of muscles and hand–eye coordination that enables a child to master tasks such as writing, grasping small objects and fastening clothing.

Flashbacks: Repeatedly reliving an earlier traumatic experience in the daytime or dreams.

Fluoxetine: An anti-depressant medication. It is a selective serotonin reuptake inhibitor (SSRI) which works by helping to regulate the levels of serotonin in the brain. Fluoxetine is used in the treatment of depression, bulimia nervosa and some anxiety disorders such as obsessive compulsive disorder. Dosage can vary from 10 mg daily to 60 mg daily, although 20 mg daily is the usual dose for an adult suffering with symptoms of depression. Fluoxetine is also approved by the European Medicines Agency, the Commission on Human Medicines and the National Institute for Clinical Excellence (UK) and the United States Food and Drug Administration (FDA) for the treatment of depression in children.

Formulation: Formulations are always used in the practice of CBT, and are the process by which the problem or problems are understood following the assessment. Formulations are presented as diagrams which explain how the various aspects which contribute to and maintain the problem fit together.

Fronto-temporal dementia: (Including Pick's disease) a type of dementia that is usually focused on the frontal lobe of the brain initially causing personality and behavioural changes (AS Fact sheet 400, Alzheimer's Society 2010).

Generalized anxiety disorder (GAD): Where the person has felt uncontrollable worry nearly every day for six months and the worry is in relation to a range of situations or issues. The worry is also excessive in relation to the event or circumstance, is distressing for the person, and their ability to function in their daily life is affected.

Genogram: A diagram representing the client's family history. It should include details of psychological and medical health.

Graded exposure: A technique often used in the treatment of simple phobias. The client is encouraged to construct a hierarchy of feared situations, and to work through them one by one, starting with the least challenging. The client must become habituated to each stage (that is, able to tolerate it without distress) before progressing to the next one.

Habituation: Through the repeated and prolonged exposure to the feared stimulus, the anxiety triggered by the fear becomes reduced to the point at which it is extinguished.

Hallucinations: Can affect all the senses and are perceived as a real experience although they don't seem to have any source. They can be in the form of auditory or voice hearing (sound), visual (sight), tactile (touch), gustatory (taste) and olfactory (smell). Voice hearing is the most common type of hallucination, and can take the form of a conversation between two voices, commenting on what the person is doing, or it can be derogatory or threatening, or warn of dangers, or command the person to do things. The voices appear to be real and so the person will then find some explanation for where the voices are coming from. They can happen over a long time and be intrusive and cause disruption, anxiety and distress.

Hallucinogens: Disrupt the interaction of nerve cells and the neurotransmitter serotonin to distort perception, and can make the user see strange shapes or vivid colours.

Heritability: The relationship between genetic variation and factors such as environment in determining the characteristics of an individual, both physical and psychological.

Heroin: A Class A drug and highly addictive with dependence developing in as brief a period as two weeks of use. Heroin is derived from the family of drugs known as opiates. It is obtained from the scored seed heads of the opium poppy and is mainly grown in Afghanistan and Pakistan. The drug is usually a reddish brown colour and can be smoked, snorted or injected.

Heroin withdrawal: Physical features related to stopping the use of heroin where the person is dependent. The features of withdrawal include: sweating, yawning, runny nose, dilated pupils, anxiety and irritability, nausea and stomach cramps, diarrhoea and vomiting, muscle aches, crawling sensations under the skin and scratching, difficulty sleeping.

Hierarchy of fears: A list of situations or events related to the feared phenomena ranked in order of the anxiety which they provoke in the person.

Higher risk drinking: Men 50+ units per week; women 35+ units per week.

Homeless outreach worker: People with a remit to engage and work with homeless people.

Homework: Work which it is agreed for the person to carry out at home and to report back on in the CBT session.

Horizontal relationships: With peers and equals and which involve cooperation, competition, support and intimacy and from which the individual derives a sense of identity and self-esteem.

Hypersomnia: Sleeping excessively compared with the person's normal pattern.

Hypervigilance: Excessive watchfulness and alertness to danger.

Hypoglycaemia: Lower than usual level of blood glucose.

Hypomania: Less pronounced than mania and, while not sufficiently severe to interrupt daily life, is nevertheless manifest in a number of ways including elevated mood, increased activity, a perceived reduced need for sleep, grandiose ideas and racing thoughts.

Hypoxia: Occurs when the body as a whole or a region of the body is deprived of oxygen, for example, it can occur when the lungs of a baby that is born too early are not developed fully.

Ideas of reference: A specific type of delusion where you feel that you are being referred to by others, for example, believing that a news reporter is commenting on your thoughts.

Increased risk drinking: Men 22–50 units per week; women 15–35 units per week.

Informal admission: The person agrees to remain in hospital voluntarily.

Informal carer: A relative or friend who provides unpaid health and social care for someone living in the community.

Insomnia: Difficulty with sleep or sleeplessness compared with the person's normal pattern.

Intensive home support: An approach adopted by community teams to enable people in crisis to be cared for in their own home rather than being admitted to hospital. Thus carers and service users receive the same level of (intensive) care at home that they would in hospital.

Intent: A statement from the person that they are going to engage in self-harm. It is a key factor in risk assessment.

Interpersonal therapy: One-to-one therapy that deals with the individual's relationship, concentrating on issues of emotional need and social interaction.

Intervention: An action intended to have a beneficial biological, social or psychological effect.

Invalidating environment: Environments where your emotions are not appropriately responded to; instead they are responded to harshly, inconsistently and/or ignored.

Labile: Rapidly changing one's mood.

Lanugo: A fine downy hair that can grow on the arms, face and trunk of a person suffering from anorexia nervosa, designed to help the body trap warm air against the skin.

Late onset drinking: Where a person begins to misuse alcohol in later life, often in response to an adverse life event

Lethargy: Lack of mental and physical activity and alertness.

Lewy body dementia: A form of dementia that is named after the tiny abnormal spherical structures that develop within neurons and lead to the degeneration of brain tissue. Symptoms can include disorientation, hallucinations and problems with planning, reasoning and problem solving (AS Fact sheet 400, Alzheimer's Society 2010).

Lithium: An effective medication often used in the treatment of bipolar disorder, both as an individual intervention (monotherapy) and also in combination with valproate to prevent relapse for relapse, as shown in the recent studies (Geddes et al. 2010). However, the use of lithium on its own for treatment of acute bipolar depression has proved not to be effective, and it is recommended to be used together with talking therapy, such as CBT, as part of a comprehensive care plan negotiated and agreed with the person.

Long-term mental health difficulties: Relate to mental illnesses that require long-term treatment and medication to maintain mental well-being. These include major psychotic illnesses such as schizophrenia and bipolar mood disorder (which often have high relapse rates).

Maintenance cycle: An understanding of the ways in which the client's problems are maintained, taking into account the relationship between thoughts, feelings and behaviours.

Mania: A manic episode can be described as a period of persistently elevated, heightened mood, consisting of euphoria and expansive goodwill, but also negative emotions such as fear, irritability and anger.

Manic depression: Formerly the term used to refer to the mental health problem of bipolar disorder.

Maudsley model: A process of family therapy designed by the London Maudsley Hospital. Its aim is to allow a reduction in parental self-blame while encouraging a familial-centred approach to out-patient treatment for anorexia nervosa in the young.

Medical intervention: The assessment of physical needs and the treatment provided by a medically qualified doctor.

Mental Health Act (1983): The MHA provides specific legal guidance defining mental disorder and a range of provisions (Sections) for the detention and treatment of people with mental health issues. A guiding rule is that the least restrictive option is required and the purpose of the Act is to ensure that appropriate care is available, and to minimize the risk of harm occurring to the person or others due to their mental ill-health.

Methadone: A heroin substitute.

Minor cognitive impairment: Where individuals have psychological symptoms similar to dementia but these are not considered severe enough to warrant a diagnosis of dementia.

Misuse of Drugs Act (1971): Provides legal regulation for and control of drugs that are banned from the UK and grades them in order of severity to the user and to the public.

Model for behaviour change: Devised by Prochaska and DiClemente (1986) and used to identify the person's level of readiness and motivation to make a meaningful change in their life. There are six stages to this model:

1 Pre-contemplation – non-recognition of the problem
2 Contemplation – recognition of there being a problem
3 Action – carrying out action to address the problem
4 Change – attempting behaviour change
5 Maintaining change – keeping the change going
6 Relapse – returning to the original behaviour.

Monoamine oxidase inhibitors (MAOIs): See **anti-depressant medication**.

Motivational interviewing (MI): A client-centred, reflective counselling style which enhances motivation for change by an interviewer helping the person clarify and resolve ambivalence about behavioural change. The goal of Motivational Interviewing is to create and amplify discrepancy between present behaviour and broader goals.

Narrative therapy: An approach to psychotherapy based on the life story of the individual, taking account of the individual's interpretations of events. The therapist works collaboratively with the client in order to help the client understand the meaning of events within the client's life, and how those events might link together. The term 'narrative therapy' is often associated with the work of Michael White and David Epston, who worked together in the 1970s and 1980s.

National census: A ten-yearly survey of households in the United Kingdom that collects a range of data including economic and social status. This is then used to plan health and social care support and local services.

National Service Framework: The *National Service Framework for Mental Health: Modern Standards and Service Models* (DoH 1999) was part of a series of standards produced by the government across all areas of health care to develop national standards across the NHS. The NSF for mental health was the second one produced, and aimed to set standards of care within the in-patient sector, while also expanding the range of services available in the community, including a commitment to introduce assertive outreach teams and crisis resolution home treatment (CRHT) teams.

Negative self-labelling: A thinking style which focused on negative personality traits.

Negative thoughts: Frequently occurring unhelpful thoughts often based on a distorted view of the evidence.

Neurofibrillary tangles: Insoluble twisted nerve fibres that mainly consist of the tau protein. In Alzheimer's disease, tau is abnormal and the microtubules in the brain cells collapse.

Neuropathology: The study of diseases of the nervous system.

No self-harm contract: An agreement drawn up by the service user and the team which prohibits self-harm, the obtaining of materials that can be used in self-harm and the immediate reporting of any self-harming behaviour.

Non-verbal communication: Sending and receiving messages without using verbal means of communication, for example, using eye contact, facial expression, posture, proximity, bodily gestures, paralanguage (sounds).

Noradrenaline: A neurotransmitter linked to the 'fight or flight' reflexes in the nervous system.

Numbing: Emotional withdrawal to avoid distressing memories.

Obsession: Experienced as intrusive thoughts, images or urges which are persistent and unwanted, and which cause significant anxiety or distress. Although the person may have insight and know these thoughts are produced by their mind, and not caused by the environment around them, and also be aware that they place an unreasonable demand or burden upon them, they are unable to prevent their occurrence (APA 2000; NCCMH 2011).

Obsessive compulsive disorder (OCD): OCD involves the presence of obsessions or compulsions, and commonly both, which the person recognizes as imposing excessive demands upon them, and impeding their everyday life. The APA (2000) suggest that a person may be experiencing OCD if the focus of the person's obsessions and compulsions requires in excess of one hour a day, although for many people these will occupy a significantly greater amount of their time.

Occupational therapist (OT): A trained healthcare professional who works with people to assess and promote effective functioning in all aspects of everyday living.

Old age: In Western society, this is believed to begin at age 60–65 or retirement from work.

Open questions: These are generalized questions and encourage the person to speak and provide a longer answer than closed questions which have a 'yes' or 'no' fixed response.

Oppositional behaviour: Confrontational or defiant behaviour, often directed at authority figures such as parents or teachers.

Oppositional defiant disorder (ODD): Is defined in DSM-IV-TR (APA 2000) as a pattern of negativistic, hostile, and defiant behavior lasting at least 6 months, during which four (or more) of the following are present:

1 often loses temper;
2 often argues with adults;
3 often actively defies or refuses to comply with adults' requests or rules;
4 often deliberately annoys people;
5 often blames others for his or her mistakes or misbehaviour;

  6 is often touchy or easily annoyed by others;

  7 is often angry and resentful;

  8 is often spiteful or vindictive.

Note: Consider a criterion met only if the behaviour occurs more frequently than is typically observed in individuals of comparable age and developmental level. See DSM-IV-TR (APA 2000) for a full definition.

Overt compulsions: Compulsions which are readily observed by others, for example, behaviours, or actions.

Palpitations: Unusually rapid, irregular or heavy heartbeat.

Panic: Frequent experience of intense fear accompanied with the physical features of anxiety.

Paroxetine: A member of the selective serotonin reuptake inhibitor (SSRI) family of anti-depressants and licensed for treatment of depression with associated anxiety. The initial dose can be increased gradually in 10 mg increments, from 20 mg to 50 mg daily. It is unwise to abruptly stop this drug and a gradual withdrawal regime should be completed over a four-week period (Levi 2007).

Patriarchal: A social structure that recognizes the father as head of the family, and men as the rightful occupants of roles of power and influence within society.

Peer group: A social group of people sharing common characteristics, for example, age, status and interests.

Persecutory delusions: A specific type of delusion or thought disorder. It is difficult to distinguish this from a plausible feeling of paranoia, it is a feeling that you are being perse-cuted or harassed.

Personality disorder: Personality disorder is a group of behaviours or characteristics which cause significant difficulty in the person's ability to function in social relationships or occu-pational settings, and is the source of much distress to the person experiencing these features.

Phobia: Phobias are anxiety-related and may be present where the person has a significant and persistent fear of a particular object or situation which is disproportionate to the actual level of risk which is present. In most cases, the person has insight and recognizes that the fear is excessive, yet feels unable to change their response.

PHQ-9: Patient Health Questionnaire. A nine-item self-administered questionnaire. It is used by GPs and other primary health care professionals to screen for symptoms of depression. It is based on DSM-IV diagnostic criteria. Copies of the questionnaire can be downloaded free at: http://www.depression-primarycare.org/clinicians/toolkits/materials/forms/phq9/ (accessed 1 August 2011).

Post-natal depression (PND): The NHS website, NHS Choices (http://www.nhs.uk/condi-tions/Postnataldepression/Pages/Symptoms.aspx, accessed 1 August 2011), defines post-natal depression as follows:

The symptoms of PND usually include one or more of the following:

- low mood for long periods of time (a week or more);
- feeling irritable for a lot of the time;
- tearfulness;
- panic attacks or feeling trapped in your life;
- difficulty concentrating;
- lack of motivation;
- lack of interest in yourself and your new baby;
- feeling lonely;

- feeling guilty, rejected or inadequate;
- feeling overwhelmed;
- feeling unable to cope;
- difficulty sleeping and feeling constantly tired;
- physical signs of tension, such as headaches, stomach pains or blurred vision;
- lack of appetite;
- reduced sex drive.

Post-traumatic stress disorder (PTSD): PTSD results from the experience of acutely traumatic and distressing life experiences. The features of this problem are typically flashbacks and nightmares, avoidance and numbing and hypervigilance.

Poverty of thought: Feeling that thinking is slowed down and difficulty generating responses to external stimuli. Among the causes include loss of motivation, negative mood or affect and inability to concentrate.

Premorbid stage: A time before there are any signs of health problems, the person is experiencing a time that is relatively stable and symptom-free (asymptomatic) and normal within the context of the individual in their setting and culture.

Primary care: Services located in the community and accessed via the family doctor, also known as the General Practitioner (GP). Examples of these services are counsellors, practice nurses, district nurses and health visitors.

Problem drinking: Alcoholics Anonymous UK regard drinking to be a problem where the physical desire to consume alcohol exceeds the person's capacity of control. An example is of a person who cannot stop drinking once they have begun, and feel unable to stop.

Problem solving: Clearly identifying the problem and then generating as wide a range of solutions as possible before considering each option in turn in terms of feasibility and appropriateness to the problem.

Prodromal stage: When the individual begins to experience a period of non-specific symptoms that may be only recognizable retrospectively and can include the following:
- depression and anxiety
- sleep problems
- poor self-care
- school work or social difficulties
- attenuated psychotic symptoms (less intense/frequent and not sustained)
- other cognitive/emotional disturbances
- low energy
- stress intolerance.

Professional support: The care provided by a range of professionally qualified workers such as nurses, social workers, physiotherapists, psychiatrists and psychologists.

Progressive muscle relaxation: The person tenses their muscles for a period of seconds, and then relaxes them progressively from their head down to their feet. The technique is improved with practice. See Figure 7.1.

Psychodynamic therapy: Psychodynamic therapy developed from the ideas of Sigmund Freud, and his concepts of the unconscious. This approach considers factors such as the client's personal history, their relationship with their parents, and the relationship between the client and the therapist. There is emphasis on understanding the way that the client's unconscious mind works to understand emotional experiences. Psychodynamic interventions tend to be of longer duration than approaches such as cognitive behavioural therapy, and may involve regular meetings between client and therapist for a year or more.

Psycho-education: Part of treatment that involves providing the client with information about their condition, in order to help them to understand what is happening to them.

Psycho-social interventions (PSI): Structured approaches that aim to alleviate the symptoms associated with a range of mental illnesses such as depression, anxiety, addiction and psychosis. Such approaches include cognitive behavioural therapy, family interventions and psycho-education.

Purging: Behaviour carried out by the person to void an excessive amount of food following a binge. This can take the form of the use of laxatives, diuretics, self-induced vomiting or a rigorous exercise regime undertaken with the specific intent of purging.

Randomized controlled trial: A randomized controlled trial (RCT) is a form of experimental research. The subjects (research participants) are randomly allocated into two groups, the Experimental group and the Control (or Comparison group). The Experimental group receives the intervention or treatment that is being tested, while the Control group receives an alternative treatment or placebo. The results of the trial are assessed by comparing the outcomes in the two different groups. The RCT is the 'gold standard' for assessing the effectiveness of an intervention because the study aims to reduce the likelihood of the outcomes being due to effects other than the intervention. (Evidence Based Nursing Practice website, accessed 25 July 2011).

Rebound symptoms: Withdrawal from benzodiazepines can produce physical symptoms, for example, in mild to moderate dependency, these might include: insomnia, sweating, anxiety and restlessness and some psychological reactions.

Recovery-based practice: Encourages a positive, hopeful and inclusive approach to mental health care. It allows all those involved to evaluate their own psychological well-being and work together to improve the lives of all those who are affected by mental health difficulties.

Relapse prevention plan: Measures to optimize the person's coping mechanisms and prevent relapse in response to setbacks or reversals.

Residential detoxification centre: An area where people live for a specific period of time while detoxifying from substance use.

Respite care: Enables carers to take a break from the pressures of their caring role. To facilitate this, the service user is cared for away from their home environment and this may involve a temporary admission to a care home or the provision of day care.

Risk: The possibility, likelihood or chance that an event may occur. The outcome of this event is not known but it can be positive or negative.

Risk assessment: A thorough assessment of the issues which may pose a risk to the safety of the individual, including risk to self, risk to others and risk from others. Wherever possible, the assessment should be conducted collaboratively with the individual concerned, and should recognize the strengths and abilities of the individual. A crisis plan should also be included so that all staff involved in the care of the individual have rapid access to an agreed management strategy.

Risk factor: Something that directly contributes to the risk event, e.g. substance use is a risk factor for self-harm.

Risk management: The process of alleviating the threat of individual risk factors so that they do not result in the risk event occurring. Also risk management may be about ensuring the harm caused by a risk event is kept at a minimum. An effective risk management plan will be multi-disciplinary and may also involve significant other people in the service user's life.

Ruminating: Pondering or deep thought, which can be experienced in depression as excessive preoccupation.

Safe drinking limits: Men: 3–4 units of alcohol per day totalling 14–21 units per week; women: 2–3 units per day totalling 14 per week; pregnant women or those trying for a baby: 1–2 units per week and avoid getting drunk.

Safety behaviour: A behaviour that is undertaken that the person believes will protect them from whatever their feared threat is. In the long run, the behaviour will stop the person from disconfirming their fears that this is in fact not the case.

Schema: This is how we psychologically view the world; schemas are broad, pervasive themes regarding oneself and one's relationship with others, developed during childhood and elaborated throughout one's lifetime, and dysfunctional to a significant degree.

Secondary care: Specialist health services which are accessed via the G P or self-referral. These include mental health and physical health services.

Section 2 of the Mental Health Act (1983): A part of the Mental Health Act (1983) under which a person can be detained within a mental health unit for up to 28 days for assessment of their mental health. The section can be ended at any time before the 28-day duration by people with appropriate authority.

Selective serotonin reuptake inhibitors (SSRIs): Anti-depressant drugs which were introduced in the U K in the early 1990s. These have fewer side effects than earlier anti-depressants and are a good choice for older patients being treated in a primary setting. They are effective for treating depression and panic disorder.

Self-harm: Any behaviour intended to hurt or harm one's self. This can include cutting, burning, taking overdoses, or drinking excessive amounts of alcohol. Self-harm may become habitual, and be used as a routine way to manage strong emotions, or may be very sporadic and only occur at times of crisis.

Simple phobias: Where the fear is towards something specific; these can include a range of things, for example, animals, the environment, the natural environment, risk and well-being, sensations and situations.

Sleep hygiene: The environment and habits which influence the quality of sleep.

Social learning theory: Behaviour learned in such a way becomes ingrained and very difficult to change.

Social Readjustment Rating Scale: Developed by Holmes and Rahe (1967) the Social Readjustment Rating Scale (S R R S) is a ranked list of stress-inducing life events.

Social withdrawal: The individual may experience difficulty in social interaction with others, they may have a flat affect and their voice may be monotone and their facial expression does not change, along with poverty of speech **(alogia)**.

Splitting: The person does not believe that good and bad attributes co-exist simultaneously and applies this view personally and to other people in: 'all or nothing' thinking. As a result, the person struggles to form enduring and trusting relationships, and often oscillates between a self-perception of being good and bad.

SSRIs: See **Selective serotonin reuptake inhibitors**.

Stages of change model: The model has been chosen as it is often used in working with addictive behaviour, for example, drugs and smoking as well as alcohol, and proceeds on the basis that successful behaviour change occurs in stages and progress will be at different rates for different people.

Standardized measures: A range of tools such as questionnaires and skills-based tests that enable health professionals to assess the severity of a patient's current symptoms. The term 'standardized' refers to the way in which the measure is devised and tested, which ensures that information gained from a measure is a reliable reflection of the patient's symptoms as compared to the general population. Examples of standardized measures include Conners' ADHD scales, the Beck Depression Inventory (Beck 1996) and the Wechsler Intelligence Scale for Children.

Stepped care: An approach to treating mental health issues whereby the least interventionist option is chosen from the range of options which are available.

Stimulants: Increase brain activity through their effect on the CNS, and can make the user feel more alert and energetic.

Stress: A condition or feeling in which the person perceives that demand is in excess of their personal and social resources at their disposal.

Stress vulnerability model: Zubin and Spring (1977) suggested that there might be a bi- genetically predisposing element to the person becoming acutely mentally unwell. However, in order for this to occur it is necessary for the person to be exposed to a trigger.

Substance misuse teams: Teams to support people with drug and alcohol issues.

Systemic therapy: The British Association for Counselling and Psychotherapy (BACP) website defines systemic therapy as 'the therapies which have, as their aim, a change in the transactional pattern of members of a system. It can be used as the generic term for family therapy and marital therapy.'

Telecare: A system of emergency response and sensors that monitor and enable people with long-term conditions to remain at home

Thiamine: Vitamin B1 and necessary for converting carbohydrates into energy for the brain and nervous system.

Thought disorders: Unusual ways of thinking, they are a disruption or disturbance to normal thought patterns; for example, passivity phenomena is a feeling that someone else has inserted a thought into their head or thought broadcasting is that thoughts are being broadcasted and that others can hear them.

Thought records: Recording thoughts which the person has, often with the intention of balancing recurrent negative thoughts with those which are more positive.

Titration of drug dosage: A gradual increase in the dosage of a drug until optimal therapeutic dose is reached, that is, no further clinical improvement is achieved through a further increase of the dose. This process ensures that the patient receives the optimum dose of medication. Side effects can also be closely monitored and taken into account when reviewing dosage.

Tolerance: The body's response to the effects of alcohol. Often as we grow older due to physical changes, our response to the same level of alcohol changes.

Transient psychosis: A brief psychotic episode lasting in duration from 1 day to 1 month.

Tricyclics: See **anti-depressant medication**.

Unconditional positive regard: Actively demonstrating a positive and non-judgemental attitude in our verbal and non-verbal communication, seeing the world through the other person's eyes and not imposing our own values and views.

Urinalysis: Testing of urine. In substance misuse, the purpose is to establish the presence of substances in the person's system.

Validation: An attempt by the clinician to get in touch with the inner emotional world of the client; involves seeking to develop an awareness of the client's feelings and attempting to understand the world from a client's perspective.

Vascular dementia: Relates to conditions such as strokes (CVA), circulatory problems, high blood pressure and small strokes that may cause a reduced oxygen supply to the brain and then brain cells die. Subsequently this might cause the signs and symptoms of dementia.

Verbal communication: Communication expressed through words.

Vertical relationships: Relationships between children and parents which provide care, nurturance and protection during the child's formative years through the parents acting as role models, teachers and providing support.

Very old age: As people have begun living longer over recent decades the term refers to people aged over 80 or approximately at or exceeding the current average lifespan. However, there are drastic regional variations for lifespan across the UK.

Vitamin B: Once thought of as a single vitamin, but research has revealed that vitamin B is a complex or group of different vitamins which exist in the same foods.

Well-being centres: Day hospitals are being re-launched as community well-being centres to emphasize their new wider role within the local community. The aims of these centres include helping people to remain in their own homes and providing specialist care for people with dementia and their carers.

Youth offending teams: Work with younger people who have come into contact with the Criminal Justice system.

REFERENCES

(APA) American Psychiatric Association (2000) *Diagnostic and Statistical Manual of Psychiatric Disorders*, text revision. Washington, DC: APA.

(AS) Alzheimer's Society (2010) *What Is Dementia?* Fact sheet number 400. London: Alzheimer's Society.

Asen, E. and Scholz, M. (2010) *Multi-Family Therapy: Concepts and Techniques*. Hove: Routledge.

Beck, J. (1996) *Cognitive Therapy: Basics and Beyond*. New York: Guilford Press.

DoH (Department of Health) (1999) *National Service Framework for Mental Health: Modern Standards and Service Models*. London: DoH.

Geddes, J.R., Goodwin, G.M., Rednell, J., Azorin, J.M., Cipriani, A., Ostacher, M.I. et al. (2010) Lithium plus valproate combination therapy versus monotherapy for relapse prevention in bipolar 1 disorder (BALANCE): a randomized open-label trial, *The Lancet*, 375: 385–95.

Holmes, T. and Rahe, R. (1967) The Social Readjustment Rating Scale, *Journal of Psychosomatic Research*, 11: 213–18.

Levi, M.I. (2007) *Basic Notes in Psychopharmacology*, 4th edn. Oxford: Radcliffe Publishing.

NCCMH (National Collaborating Centre for Mental Health) (2011) *Common Mental Health Disorders: Identification and Pathways to Care*. National Clinical Guideline Number 123. London: NICE.

NICE (National Institute for Health and Clinical Excellence) (2005) Clinical Guidance 31, *Obsessive Compulsive Disorder (OCD) and Body Dysmorphic Disorder (BDD)*. London: NICE.

Prochaska, J.O. and DiClemente, C.C. (1986) Toward a comprehensive model of change, in W. R. Miller and N. Heather (eds) *Treating Addictive Behaviors: Processes of Change*. New York: Plenum Press.

Richardson, G. and Wyatt, A. (2010) CAMHS in context, in G. Richardson, I. Partridge, and J. Barrett, (eds) *Child and Adolescent Mental Health Services: An Operational Handbook*. 2nd edn. London: RCPsych Publications.

WHO (World Health Organization) (2001) *Audit: The Alcohol Use Disorders Identification Test: Guidelines for Use in Primary Care*. 2nd edn. Geneva: WHO.

Zubin, J. and Spring, B. (1977) Vulnerability: a new view on schizophrenia, *Journal of Abnormal Psychology*, 86: 103–26.

Index

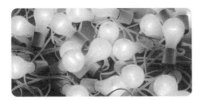
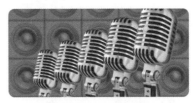
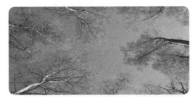
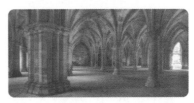
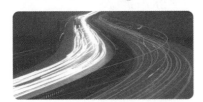
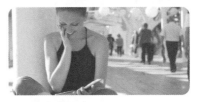
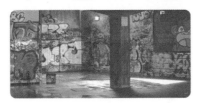

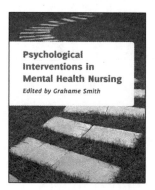

PSYCHOLOGICAL INTERVENTIONS IN MENTAL HEALTH NURSING

Grahame Smith

9780335244164 (Paperback)
April 2012

eBook also available

"This book provides excellent foundations in common psychological interventions that are used in mental health and other fields of nursing ... Each chapter uses a scenario, which helps to apply the concepts to the real world of providing healthcare. This is reinforced by the robust manner in which the text signposts readers to examples which they may use or test out in their day to day practice of mental health nursing."
Paul Barber, Senior Lecturer, University of Chester, UK

Key features:

- Underpinned by the NMC's (2010) standards for pre-registration nursing education
- Full of case studies, practical tips and a full evidence base
- Written by experts in the field who all have extensive experience in the use of psychological interventions within the clinical arena

www.openup.co.uk

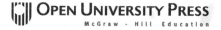

OPEN UNIVERSITY PRESS
McGraw - Hill Education